DI308122

Inside—Find the Answers to These Questions and More

- ☑ What are the seven general warning symptoms of cancer? (See page 19.)

- ☑ Are there specific foods I should eat to reduce my cancer risk? (See page 48.)

- ☑ I know exercise is good for me, but it can't prevent cancer . . . can it? (See page 140.)

- ☑ Can eating tomatoes really reduce the risk of prostate cancer? (See page 110.)

- ☑ Will taking vitamin E reduce my risk of getting prostate cancer? (See page 68.)

- ☑ Can soybeans and flaxseed oil reduce my risk of breast cancer? (See pages 111 and 120.)

- ☑ Can foods high in vitamin C provide extra insurance against cancer? (See page 89.)

- ☑ Does green tea have a general anticancer effect? (See page 115.)

- ☑ Can garlic reduce my risk of colon cancer? (See page 119.)

- ☑ It seems like just about everything causes cancer these days! What carcinogens should I *really* worry about? (See page 152.)

THE NATURAL PHARMACIST Library

Arthritis

Diabetes

Echinacea and Immunity

Feverfew and Migraines

Garlic and Cholesterol

Ginkgo and Memory

Heart Disease Prevention

Herbs

Illnesses and Their Natural Remedies

Kava and Anxiety

Menopause

PMS

Reducing Cancer Risk

Saw Palmetto and the Prostate

St. John's Wort and Depression

Vitamins and Supplements

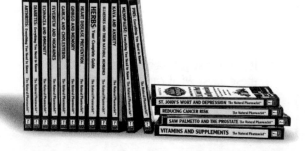

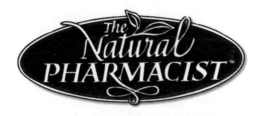

Everything You Need to Know About

Reducing
Cancer Risk

Richard Harkness, Pharm., FASCP

Series Editors

Steven Bratman, M.D.

David Kroll, Ph.D.

Prima
HEALTH

A DIVISION OF PRIMA PUBLISHING

Visit us online at www.thenaturalpharmacist.com

Warning—Disclaimer

This book is not intended to provide medical advice and is sold with the understanding that the publisher and the authors are not liable for the misconception or misuse of information provided. The authors and Prima Publishing shall have neither liability nor responsibility to any person or entity with respect to any loss, damage, or injury caused or alleged to be caused directly or indirectly by the information contained in this book or the use of any products mentioned. Readers should not use any of the products discussed in this book without the advice of a medical professional.

The Food and Drug Administration has not approved the use of any of the natural treatments discussed in this book. This book, and the information contained herein, has not been approved by the Food and Drug Administration.

All products mentioned in this book are trademarks of their respective companies.

Pseudonyms have been used throughout to protect the privacy of the individuals involved.

PRIMA HEALTH and colophon are trademarks of Prima Communications, Inc.
THE NATURAL PHARMACIST is a trademark of Prima Communications, Inc.

Library of Congress Cataloging-in-Publication Data

Harkness, Richard.
    Reducing cancer risk / Richard Harkness.
      p.   cm. — (The natural pharmacist)
    Includes bibliographical references and index.
    ISBN 0-7615-1557-7
    1. Cancer—Prevention.   2. Dietary supplements.   3. Cancer—Chemoprevention.
I. Title.   II. Series.
RC268.H29 1999
616.99'405—dc21

                                 98-48205
                                     CIP

00 01 02 03 HH 10 9 8 7 6 5 4 3
Printed in the United States of America

Visit us online at www.primahealth.com

Contents

What Makes This Book Different?

The interest in natural medicine has never been greater. According to the National Association of Chain Drug Stores, 65 million Americans are using natural supplements, and the number is growing! Yet it is hard for the consumer to find trustworthy sources for balanced information about this emerging field. Why? Frankly, natural medicine has had a checkered history. From snake oil potions sold at the turn of the century to those books, magazines, and product catalogs that hype miracle cures today, this is a field where exaggerated claims have been the norm. Proponents of natural medicine have tended to abuse science, treating it more as a marketing tool than a means of discovering the truth.

But there is truth to be found. Studies of vitamins, minerals, and other food supplements have been with us since these nutritional substances were first discovered, and the level and quality of this science has grown dramatically in the last 20 years. Herbal medicine has been neglected in the United States, but in Europe, this, the oldest of all healing arts, has been the subject of tremendous and ongoing scientific interest.

At present, for a number of herbs and supplements, it is possible to give reasonably scientific answers to the questions: How well does this work? How safe is it? What types of conditions is it best used for?

The Natural Pharmacist series is designed to cut through the hype and tell you what we know and what we don't know about popular natural treatments. These books are more conservative than any others available, more honest about the weaknesses of natural approaches, more fair in their comparisons of natural and conventional treatments. You won't find any miracle cures here, but you will discover useful options that can help you become healthier.

Why Choose Natural Treatments?

Although the science behind natural medicine continues to grow, this is still a much less scientifically validated field than conventional medicine. You might ask, "Why should I resort to an herb that is only partly proven, when I could take a drug with solid science behind it?" There are at least three good reasons to consider natural alternatives.

First, some herbs and supplements offer benefits that are not matched by any conventional drug. Vitamin E is a good example. It appears to help prevent prostate cancer, a benefit that no standard medication can claim. Also, vitamin E almost certainly helps prevent heart disease. While there are standard drugs that also prevent heart disease, vitamin E works differently and may be able to complement many of the other approaches.

Another example is the herb milk thistle. Studies strongly suggest that this herb can protect the liver from injury. There is no pill or tablet your doctor can prescribe to do the same.

Even if the science behind some of these treatments is less than perfect, when the risks are low and the possible benefit high, a treatment may be worth trying. It is a little-known fact that for many conventional treatments the science is less than perfect as well, and physicians must balance uncertain benefits against incompletely understood risks.

A second reason to consider natural therapies is that some may offer benefits comparable to those of drugs with fewer side effects. The herb St. John's wort is a good example. Reasonably strong scientific evidence suggests that this herb is an effective treatment for mild to moderate depression, while producing fewer side effects on average than conventional medications. Saw palmetto for benign enlargement of the prostate, ginkgo for relieving symptoms and perhaps slowing the progression of Alzheimer's disease, and glucosamine for osteoarthritis are other examples. This is not to say that herbs and supplements are completely harmless—they're not—but for most the level of risk is quite low.

Finally, there is a philosophical point to consider. For many people, it "feels" better to use a treatment that comes from nature instead of from a laboratory. Just as you might rather wear all-cotton clothing than polyester, or look at a mountain landscape rather than the skyscrapers of a downtown city, natural treatments may simply feel more compatible with your view of life. We can quibble endlessly about just what "natural" means and whether a certain treatment is "actually" natural or not, but such arguments are beside the point. The difference is in the feeling, and feelings matter. In fact, having a good feeling about taking an herb may lead you to use it more consistently than you would a prescription drug.

Of course, at times synthetic drugs may be necessary and even lifesaving. But on many other occasions it may be quite reasonable to turn to an herb or supplement instead of a drug.

To make good decisions you need good information. Unfortunately, while hundreds of books on alternative medicine are published every year, many are highly misleading. The phrase "studies prove" is often used when the studies in question are so small or so badly conducted that they prove nothing at all. You may even find that the "data" from other books come from studies with petri dishes and not real people!

You can't even assume that books written by well-known authors are scientifically sound. Many of these authors rely on secondary writers, leading to a game of "telephone," where misconceptions are passed around from book to book. And there's a strong tendency to exaggerate the power of natural remedies, whitewashing them with selective reporting.

THE NATURAL PHARMACIST series gives you the balanced information you need to make informed decisions about your health needs. Setting a new, high standard of accuracy and objectivity, these books take a realistic look at the herbs and supplements you read about in the news. You will encounter both favorable and unfavorable studies in these pages and will learn about both the benefits and the risks of natural treatments.

THE NATURAL PHARMACIST series is the source you can trust.

Steven Bratman, M.D.
David Kroll, Ph.D.

Introduction

*T*he *Natural Pharmacist Guide to Reducing Cancer Risk* is for people who have never had cancer as well as those who have survived the disease. Everyone wishes to stay cancer-free, and cancer survivors wish to avoid a recurrence or another cancer.

And there is *very* good news about preventing cancer, which we'll get to in chapter 1. First, here's some background. Our modern understanding of the biology of the cancer process (carcinogenesis) has led not only to new potential treatments, but also to better possible preventive measures. Perhaps more so with cancer than with any other disease, an ounce of prevention really is worth a pound of cure.

Traditional treatments include surgery, radiation, chemotherapy, and biological therapy. Treatment leads to cures in over 50% of patients, mostly due to surgery.[1] This fact may seem pleasantly surprising, but it's still not hearty news. And to become survivors, patients may have to undergo horrendous, long-term suffering caused by the very treatments designed to heal them. (The first three treatments above are often wryly called cut, burn, and poison.)

Prevention now means more than merely avoiding cancer-causing agents (carcinogens). It includes practical ways to actively lower our risk and screen for early cancer detection. There are two types of preventive strategies: primary and secondary.

Primary prevention includes proactive measures to remain cancer-free, such as smoke cessation, sun avoidance, eating properly, exercising, and chemoprevention (referring primarily to the use of specific synthetic or natural agents to prevent cancer). Secondary prevention consists of detecting already forming cancer as early as possible and treating it effectively. We will attend to both, with our primary focus on the much more desirable goal of primary prevention: stopping cancer from getting a foothold to begin with.

Natural chemopreventive agents are found in many foods, herbs, and nutritional supplements. Using diet and nutritional supplements to stop cancer in its tracks (by short-circuiting the underlying carcinogenesis process) is not far-fetched. We routinely prevent heart and kidney disease and stroke by controlling high blood pressure (the underlying process) with medications. Chemoprevention is not yet widely established in clinical practice, but it's a current hot research topic and studies are showing great promise.

Screening, a secondary preventive tactic, is designed to detect cancer early in individuals without symptoms. The earlier it's found, the more likely it can be eradicated. Screening has become more popular as more tests have been developed that are quick, safe, and inexpensive. Screenings for colon, cervical, and breast cancer have saved countless lives. Genetic screening for high-risk individuals will burgeon as more cancer-predisposing genes are identified. We will have to deal with ethical dilemmas in this arena.

The Good News: You Can Cut Your Cancer Risk

Despite some grim statistics, the dark visitant called cancer need not inevitably come calling. It often needs your help to slink through the door.

You can cut your cancer risk 60 to 70% *by what you choose to do.* That's the bright consensus of an international panel recently convened by the American Institute for Cancer Research and the World Cancer Research Fund.[2] The panel found four key ways you can keep cancer away: Eat the right foods, exercise, watch your weight, and don't smoke. The experts reviewed diet and cancer findings from over 4,500 studies to reach this consensus.

The Natural Pharmacist Guide to Reducing Cancer Risk analyzed the newest research findings to discover other important ways to reduce your risk even more, including the use of nutritional supplements that appear to have anticancer activity. You can start using this information immediately.

The anticancer lifestyle adds a bonus—protection from heart disease, high blood pressure, diabetes, and many other serious chronic ailments.

At today's frenetic pace, sticking to a healthful lifestyle is easier said than done, but many others have done it and you can, too. People often wait to act until faced with cancer or some other life-menacing illness. Act proactively and you might never have to greet that day of reckoning.

For some people, easing into a more healthful lifestyle one step at a time may work best for creating the mindset needed to eventually jump in completely. You may not be able to do all the recommended things at once. Do one, then add another, as your situation and level of commitment permit. Each element alone may provide a significant benefit, but the comprehensive "holistic" approach should be the goal. That first step is the hardest. Once you get going, it becomes a habit. And by that time, you'll feel so good you won't want to stop!

So a large measure of control is yours for the taking. With reliable, balanced information and some effort, you and your family stand an excellent chance of remaining cancer-free. And that's truly good news. This book shows you how.

About Cancer

C ancer costs are staggering financially, both to the individual and society. According to the National Cancer Institute, cancer costs $107 billion a year: $37 billion in direct medical costs, $11 billion in morbidity costs (lost productivity), and $59 billion in mortality (dying) costs. Breast, lung, and prostate cancers account for over half of direct medical costs. As of 1994, about 18% of Americans under age 65 had no health insurance, and about 14% of older persons had only Medicare coverage.

Incidence

Cancer is the second major cause of death (next to heart disease) in the United States, claiming the lives of more than half a million Americans a year out of the nearly 1.4 million who get the disease. The probability of getting cancer increases with age. Two-thirds of all cases occur in people over age 65.[1]

The American Cancer Society estimates that one in two men and one in three women will face cancer during their lifetimes. Most cancers require several years to develop, so it's never too early to start practicing protective prevention.

Major cancers include prostate (male), breast (female), lung, colon and rectum, gynecologic areas (uterus, cervix, ovary), urinary bladder, stomach, oral cavity and pharynx, leukemia, lymphomas, pancreas, and skin (see table 1).

What Is Cancer?

Cancer is an invasive, uncontrolled replication of abnormal body cells. These aberrant cells crowd out and injure

Cancer is the second major cause of death in the United States.

or destroy healthy cells, eventually causing enough damage to threaten the function of critical organ systems. The approximately 150 different types of cancer share this common blueprint. When doctors and scientists talk about cancer, they may speak of a *malignant* (harmful or invasive) *neoplasm* (a new, abnormal growth or tumor). As we talk about cancer throughout this book, it will help to know some specific terms.

Some Specific Terms

Cancers are broadly classified as carcinomas, sarcomas, leukemias, or lymphomas. A *carcinoma* arises in epithelial tissue, which covers the skin and lines body cavities and organs. A *sarcoma* occurs in connective tissue such as muscle or bone and the linings of organs. *Leukemia* develops in blood-forming tissues such as the spleen and bone marrow. A *lymphoma* forms in the lymphatic system,

Table 1. Cancer Incidence (Deaths)*, 2

Male		Female	
Prostate	41 (14)	Breast	31 (17)
Lung	13 (32)	Lung	13 (25)
Colon and rectum	9 (9)	Colon and rectum	11 (10)
Urinary	7 (5)	Uterus	6 (3)
Leukemia, lymphomas	6 (9)	Leukemia, lymphomas	6 (8)
Melanoma (skin)	3 (2)	Urinary	4 (3)
Oral	3 (2)	Ovary	4 (6)
Pancreas	2 (5)	Cervix uteri	3 (2)
Stomach	2 (3)	Melanoma (skin)	3 (1)
All other	14 (19)	Pancreas	2 (5)
Oral	2 (1)	All other	15 (20)

*For example, in males, prostate cancer accounts for 41% of all cancers and a death rate of 14% of all cancers.

which filters out harmful bacteria, viruses, and dead cells. Types of lymphoma include Hodgkin's disease, non-Hodgkin's lymphoma, and Burkitt's lymphoma.

Metastasis occurs when cancer cells in one part of the body break loose and spread to other parts through the blood or lymphatic systems.

In situ, Latin for "in position," refers to cancer that has not yet spread—it is localized and at an early stage. Most such cancers are curable if corralled before they progress to invasive cancer. The importance of screening, as we'll see in detail later, is that it can catch cancers at this early stage.

Most cancers require several years to develop, so it's never too early to start practicing protective prevention.

What Causes Cancer?

Cancer is a genetic disease because damaged genes that control cell replication can either be inherited or acquired during a person's own lifetime. Like most diseases, cancer develops through an interaction between genetics and environment, with the tilt toward environment. Most of the cell mutations that lead to cancer result from internal DNA errors and/or exposure to cancer-causing agents (carcinogens) in the environment. It's estimated that about 60% of human cancer can be clearly traced to environmental or lifestyle factors.[3]

However, the meaning of "environmental" in this regard has become muddled. A widespread, distorted view is that it refers to industrial pollution, toxic wastes, and various chemicals dispersed in the environment. In fact, the best estimate is that only 2% of cancer deaths are related to pollution of all types.

Much more important "environmental" cancer causes are personal or lifestyle factors, of which cigarette smoking and improper diet lead the pack by many furlongs. There are also naturally occurring carcinogens in food plants as well as carcinogens that come into being when food is cooked. Because most cancers have environmental roots, they are theoretically preventable (see table 2).

Sixty percent of human cancer can be clearly traced to environmental or lifestyle factors.

Different populations experience unique cancer risks. People who move about (migrants) tend to adopt the cancer pattern of their new environments, sometimes within decades (as seen in migrants to Australia); or sometimes within generations, as seen with breast cancer in Japanese migrants to the United States.

Table 2. Ranking the Risks

Risk Factors for Cancer	% Deaths from
Tobacco/smoking	30
Diet, obesity	30
Sedentary lifestyle	5
Occupational factors	5
Family history of cancer	5
Viruses, biological agents	5
Perinatal factors, growth	5
Sexual/reproductive patterns	3
Alcohol (ethanol) use	3
Socioeconomic status	3
Environmental pollution	2
Ionizing, ultraviolet radiation (e.g., sun exposure)	2
Prescriptions, medical procedures	1
Salt, food additives, contaminants	1

Adapted from US News & World Report *(December 2, 1996) 121:22, 19,* from basic data: Harvard University School of Public Health.

Subgroups in a larger community (such as Mormons, Seventh Day Adventists, and African Americans in some parts of the United States) may have unique cancer risks apart from the general population, because of lifestyle factors unique to the group. The available evidence all points to the importance of environment in cancer risk.[4]

How Does Cancer Form in the Body?

A single cell is the unit of life of all living organisms. Within each cell is a nucleus containing 23 duplicate pairs of threadlike structures called *chromosomes.* The chromosomes contain genes made up of *DNA* (deoxyribonucleic acid). DNA is the chemical basis of heredity and the carrier of genetic information, which children inherit from their parents and, in turn, pass on to their children.

Division of healthy cells is a normal process the body uses to grow and to replace diseased or dying cells. Just before a cell divides, each chromosome forms a replica of itself. One set of chromosomes moves into the new cell. When cell division is done, the newly duplicated cell has a full set of chromosome pairs identical to that of the parent cell. The orderly process continues: Two cells become four, four become eight, and so on.

The Two-Hit Theory

Cancer develops through an accumulation of genetic changes within a cell. In the "two-hit" theory, the progression of a cell to cancer requires *initiation* (the first hit) followed by *promotion* (the second hit).[5]

A mutation is the first hit (initiation). It results from damage to DNA instructions. The body is bombarded by

The two-hit theory: The progression of a cell to cancer requires both initiation (the first hit) followed by promotion (the second hit).

thousands of initiation events daily, but our cells are amazingly resilient. Most damage is repaired, but over the course of a lifetime, the risk increases that a mutation may escape our normal DNA repair tools. Genes that carry this misprinted code pass on defective biologic instructions to future generations of cells. Damaged DNA can result from random internal errors in replication or repair (nature deals in volume), or exposure to environmental carcinogens such as cigarette smoke. A mutated gene can be inherited. For example, one of two important genes that control cell growth may mutate. The damaged form of this gene is then passed along to an offspring. Often, this mutation is "silent" in that it does not necessarily lead to cancer. However, inheritance of this one mutation makes it easier to acquire a second mutation from environmental factors. Numerous mutations may occur along the way toward cancer.

A flawed cell is vulnerable to becoming cancerous. Still, one more step is necessary. To actually become cancerous, the cell must suffer a second hit (promotion). Promoters stimulate cell growth and allow mutations to start working. Hormones often unwittingly play the role of promoter. Intended by nature to keep certain normal cells healthy, they may act on mutated cells to push them into uncontrolled growth: Examples include androgens (male sex hormones) that are linked to prostate cancer and estrogen which is linked to breast and uterine cancers.

Another factor is free radicals. These renegade molecules can be formed from environmental toxins as well as from normally desirable substances such as oxygen. The unpaired electrons in free radicals are unstable and aggressively combine with other essential molecules, damaging them. Ordinarily, the body's natural antioxidants neutralize free radicals. In some cases, though, free radicals ravage out of control and deplete stores of our own antioxidants, a process that may help jumpstart cancer. We'll look at the role of antioxidants in detail later when we discuss nutritional supplements.

Because it takes a long time for most premalignant lesions to become fully cancerous, much current research on prevention is aimed at the promotion stage.

Initiation is a quick, permanent hit, while promotion is a slower, progressive process that can stretch over years. Because it takes a long time for most premalignant lesions to become fully cancerous, much current research on prevention is aimed at the promotion stage.

The Beginning of Cancer

The entire process of initiation, promotion, and progression by which healthy cells turn into cancer cells is called *carcinogenesis*. It takes a while. Healthy cells don't go bad overnight.

But if enough mutations accumulate and the right promoters are present, eventually the orderly process of cell

division we spoke of earlier turns into a clutter of cellular confusion.[6] Genes that tell cells to stop dividing get stuck in the "on" position; instructions that prevent runaway growth get scrambled; systems that block or repair mutations become disabled; molecular guards fall asleep at critical checkpoints; and signals begin to fail that would normally tell cells to die when they have accumulated too great a burden of DNA damage. These bad cells that would ordinarily die now become "immortalized." The entire system of checks and balances runs amok.

> On a positive note, at each step along the lengthy, winding road to cancer, we're finding bridges of vulnerability that can be blocked with natural cancer-preventive agents.

Still, roaming cancer cells must evade the immune system's macrophage white blood cells and other roving biologic commandos whose job is to find and destroy molecular marauders. However, the immune system may not be operating at its peak due to stress, other debilitating diseases, or a subpar diet. Some cancers may overpower even a healthy immune system. And, since cancer cells arise from our own previously normal cells, the immune system may not always recognize them as foes.

On a positive note, at each step along the lengthy, winding road to cancer, we're finding bridges of vulnerability that can be blocked with natural cancer-preventive agents.

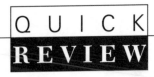

QUICK REVIEW

- Cancer is second only to heart disease among major causes of death in the United States.

  Breast and prostate cancer are the most frequently occurring cancers, while lung cancer claims the most deaths in both men and women, followed by breast cancer in women.

- Cancer is an invasive, uncontrolled replication of abnormal body cells. Cancer *in situ* (in position) has not spread to other parts of the body. Most cancers are curable if detected and treated at this stage.

- Sixty percent of human cancer can be clearly traced to environmental or lifestyle factors.

  Like most diseases, cancer develops through an interaction between genetics and environment, with the tilt toward environment.

- According to the "two-hit" theory, the progression to cancer requires initiation (the first hit) followed by promotion (the second hit).

Initiation is the result of damage to the DNA in a gene, which passes the faulty instructions on to subsequent cells.

Promoters include environmental carcinogens such as cigarette smoke and the body's own sex hormones.

- Because it takes a long time for most premalignant lesions to become fully cancerous, much current research on prevention is aimed at the promotion stage.

T W O

Assess Your Risk

S ome people are more at risk for cancer than others. Knowing where you stand can help you plan your cancer prevention strategy.

Lifetime risk refers to your chance of getting cancer during your life. In the United States, for example, lifetime risk for men is one in two chances and for women it is one in three. *Relative risk* refers to your chances of getting a particular cancer, and has to do with specific risk factors linked to that type of cancer. Different people have different relative risks because of their individual traits or exposures. Smokers, for example, are ten times more likely to get lung cancer than nonsmokers. Something that increases your relative risk is called a risk factor. Most risk factors are not as powerful as smoking. For instance, women with a first-degree family history of breast cancer (mother, sister, or daughter) are only twice as likely to get breast cancer as women with no such family history. However, this is still obviously quite serious.

11

Assessing Your Relative Risks

Assessing your risk factors helps you determine where to put your emphasis in choosing anticancer foods, nutri-

tional supplements, and screening tests for early detection. Some of the risk factors for the cancers listed below can't be altered, but others can, and we'll see how in detail in chapter 3. Let's look at the risk factors for each of several major cancers.[1] The primary source for the information in this chapter is the *American Cancer Society: Cancer Facts & Figures—1998.*

Lifetime risk of cancer for men is one in two chances and for women it is one in three.

Breast Cancer Risk Factors

For women, breast cancer risk factors include personal or family history of breast cancer; biopsy-confirmed atypical hyperplasia (excessive cell proliferation or reproduction); early menarche (first menstrual period before age 12); late menopause; recent use of oral contraceptives or post-menopausal estrogens; never having children or having the first live birth at a late age (over age 30). Risk also appears to correlate with the amount of fat in the diet, though this has not been firmly established.

Other possible risk factors being studied are alcohol use, weight gain, sedentary lifestyle, induced abortion, and pesticide/chemical exposure. Current research is trying to unlock the role of the breast cancer susceptibility genes BRCA1 and BRCA2.

If you have risk factors for breast cancer, the following topics will be of special interest: Essential Screening Information for Breast Cancer, and Breast Self-Exam in chapter 3; Fat and Cancer, and Monounsaturated Fats and Breast Cancer in chapter 4; the topics on vitamin E, vitamin C, and vitamin D in chapter 5; the topics on tomatoes, soybeans, flaxseed oil, melatonin, rosemary, and tangerines in chapter 6; and Exercise and Weight Control: A Foundation for Good Health, and Alcohol in chapter 7.

Prostate Cancer Risk Factors

For men, risk factors for prostate cancer include age (over 75% of all prostate cancers occur in men past age 65); race (African Americans are at highest risk); genetics (5 to 10% of cases may be inherited); and dietary fat. Prostate cancer is common in North America and northwestern Europe, and rare in Asia, Africa, and South America.

Smokers are ten times more likely to get lung cancer than nonsmokers.

If you have risk factors for prostate cancer, the following topics will be of special interest: Prostate Cancer in chapter 3; Fat and Cancer in chapter 4; the topics on vitamin E, selenium, vitamin C, and vitamin D in chapter 5; and the topics on tomatoes, soybeans, and melatonin in chapter 6.

Colorectal Cancer Risk Factors

Risk factors for colorectal cancer (cancer of the colon and rectum) include personal or family history of colorectal cancer or polyps, and inflammatory bowel disease. Other possible risk factors are sedentary lifestyle, high-fat and/or low-fiber diet, and not eating enough fruits and vegetables.

If you have risk factors for colorectal cancer, the following topics will be of special interest: Colorectal Cancer in chapter 3; Fat and Cancer, Fiber: What You Can't Digest Can Be Good for You and The Food Guide Pyramid Is Your Map to Healthful Eating in chapter 4; the topics on vitamin E, selenium, beta-carotene, vitamin C, folic acid, vitamin D, and calcium in chapter 5; the topics on tomatoes, soybeans, green tea, garlic and onion, turmeric and curcumin, and milk and dairy foods in chapter 6; and Exercise and Weight Control: A Foundation for Good Health in chapter 7.

Risk factors for breast cancer include family history, early first menstrual period, late menopause, recent use of estrogen, never having children or having the first live birth after age 30.

Cervical Cancer Risk Factors

Risk factors for cervical cancer include first intercourse at an early age; multiple sexual partners (or partners who have had multiple sexual partners); and cigarette smoking. The sexual behavior risks are linked to infections such as that from the human papilloma virus.

If you have risk factors for cervical cancer, the following topics will be of special interest: Cervical Cancer in chapter 3; the topics on vitamin C and folic acid in chapter 5; the topics on blue-green algae and ellagic acid in chapter 6; and Smoking/Tobacco, and Viral Infections in chapter 7.

Endometrial (Uterine) Cancer Risk Factors

For the most common form of endometrial (uterine) cancer, exposure to estrogen is the major risk factor (for example, estrogen replacement therapy or ERT). Using hormone replacement therapy (HRT), in which progesterone is combined with estrogen, may offset the risk of estrogen. Other risks include use of the cancer drug tamoxifen; early menarche (before age 12); late menopause; never having children; history of failure to ovulate; infertility; diabetes; gallbladder disease; hypertension; and obesity.

Pregnancy and the use of oral contraceptives appear to protect against endometrial cancer.

In the less common type of endometrial cancer, an estrogen link has not been proven. This form is more aggressive and has a poorer prognosis.

If you have risk factors for endometrial cancer, the following topics will be of special

Risk factors for colorectal cancer include sedentary lifestyle, high-fat and/or low-fiber diet, and not eating enough fruits and vegetables.

interest: Endometrial (Uterine) Cancer in chapter 3; the Food Guide Pyramid Is Your Map to Healthful Eating in chapter 4; the topic on beta-carotene in chapter 5; the topic on soybeans in chapter 6; and Exercise and Weight Control: A Foundation for Good Health in chapter 7.

Ovarian Cancer Risk Factors

Risk factors for ovarian cancer include age (risk peaks in the 80s); never having children: breast cancer or family history of breast or ovarian cancer (mutations in genes BRCA1 or BRCA2 have been noted); and hereditary non-polyposis colon cancer. Industrialized countries, with the exception of Japan, have the highest incidence rates.

Pregnancy and the use of oral contraceptives may reduce the risk of developing ovarian cancer.

If you have risk factors for ovarian cancer, the following topic will be of special interest: Ovarian Cancer in chapter 3.

Oral Cavity and Pharynx Cancer Risk Factors

Risk factors for cancers of the mouth and pharynx include smoking (cigarette, cigar, and pipe), smokeless tobacco, and excessive alcohol consumption.

If you have risk factors for these cancers, the following topics will be of special interest: Oral Cavity and Pharynx Cancer in chapter 3; the topic on beta-carotene in chapter 5; the topic on blue-green algae in chapter 6; and Smoking/Tobacco, and Alcohol in chapter 7.

Skin Cancer Risk Factors

In general, skin cancer risk factors include family history; excessive exposure to sunlight or other ultraviolet (UV) radiation (such as tanning beds); occupational exposure to coal tar, pitch, creosote, arsenic compounds, or radium.

For melanoma (the most deadly type of skin cancer), risk factors include family history of melanoma; three or more blistering sunburns before age 20; three or more summers as a teen spent working outdoors; exposures to intense sun; fair skin or hair; blue eyes; the presence of several large, brown moles at birth; and more than 25 moles larger than $1/16$ of an inch across.

For the other two types of skin cancer, squamous cell and basal cell carcinoma (see chapter 3), risk factors include decades of sun exposures; fair skin; freckles; and blue eyes.

If you have risk factors for skin cancer, the following topics will be of special interest: Skin Cancer, and Skin Self-Exam in chapter 3; the topic on vitamin C in chapter 5; the topics on bromelain, grapes, ellagic acid, and white birch tree in chapter 6; and Excessive Sun Exposure in chapter 7.

Lung Cancer Risk Factors

Cigarette smoking presents the greatest risk for lung cancer. Other risk factors include exposure to industrial agents such as arsenic; certain organic chemicals; radon; asbestos; radiation exposure; air pollution; tuberculosis; and secondhand smoke.

If you have risk factors for lung cancer, the following topics will be of special interest: Lung Cancer in chapter 3; the topics on selenium, beta-carotene, and vitamin C in chapter 5; the topics on bromelain, ellagic acid, and apples in chapter 6; and Smoking/Tobacco, and Radon in chapter 7.

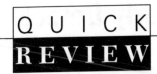

- In the United States one in two men will develop cancer over their lifetimes, while one in three women will develop cancer.
- Different cancers are associated with specific risk factors.

  Smokers are ten times more likely than nonsmokers to get lung cancer.

  Women with a first-degree family history of breast cancer (mother, sister, or daughter) are twice as likely to get breast cancer as women without a family history of cancer.
- Assessing your risks helps you determine where to put your emphasis in choosing anticancer foods, nutritional supplements, and screening tests for early detection.

Use Preventive Screenings for Early Detection

Detecting cancer early dramatically increases the likelihood of effective treatment and cure, thus preventing full-blown cancer. Preventive screenings and self-examinations are designed to detect already-forming cancers at an early stage, before they produce obvious symptoms and when there is a good possibility the cancer can be stopped. Detecting cancer early like this is part of secondary prevention. *Primary* prevention means actually stopping the cancer from developing in the first place. This is obviously even more desirable, and will be the subject of much of the rest of the book.[1] But primary prevention is not perfect. It lowers your risk of cancer but does not reduce it to zero. So don't put so much confidence in primary prevention that you dismiss the benefits of secondary preventive screenings to catch cancer early. The chief source for the information in this chapter is the *American Cancer Society: Cancer Facts & Figures—1998.*

Cancers that are found through screenings make up about half of all new cancer cases. Regularly performed self-exams for breast and skin cancer can catch many more early cancers. (The methods are detailed in this chapter.) The 5-year relative survival rate for these cancers is about 80%; regular screenings could increase that success rate to over 95%.

Primary prevention means actually stopping the cancer from developing in the first place.

Today, more people are surviving cancer than ever before. Early in the century, few patients lived very long after diagnosis. By the 1930s, about 1 in 4 individuals were alive 5 years after treatment. Currently, 4 of 10 patients are alive 5 years later. The *relative 5-year survival rate,* based on averaging, is a standard monitoring measurement that includes those who are disease-free, in remission, or still under treatment. Patients who survive 5 years are generally regarded as cured. When adjusted for other factors such as accidents, heart disease, and other diseases, the relative 5-year survival rate is 58% for all cancers. The earlier you catch cancer, the better your chances of beating it.

Cancer's Seven General Warning Symptoms

Change in bowel or bladder habits.
A sore that doesn't heal.
Unusual bleeding or discharge.
Thickening or lump in breast or elsewhere.
Indigestion or difficulty in swallowing.
Obvious change in a wart or mole.
Nagging cough or hoarseness.

Keeping in mind cancer's seven *general* warning symptoms can help you catch the disease in an early stage. Simply remember the mnemonic term CAUTION, by combining the first letter of each item in the preceding list.

The rest of this chapter looks at essential screening information for cancers of the breast, prostate, colon and rectum, cervix, endometrium (uterus), ovary, oral cavity and pharynx, skin, and lung. Genetic screening may be an option if you have a family history of certain cancers.

Essential Screening Information for Breast Cancer

The earliest sign of breast cancer is usually an abnormality that neither you nor your health care examiner may be able to feel, but may be detected by a mammogram. Later, symptoms may include a breast lump, thickening, swelling, distortion, or tenderness; skin irritation or dimpling; or nipple pain, scaliness, or retraction. Breast pain is commonly due to benign conditions, and is not usually the first symptom of breast cancer. Men can also get breast cancer, though it is much rarer than in women.

Screening

Mammography can find breast abnormalities at an early stage, before symptoms develop. Early detection increases your treatment options. The American Cancer Society's guidelines stress mammography and physical examinations.

Most breast lumps are not cancerous, but only a physician can tell. When a suspicious lump or area is identified on a mammogram, diagnostic mammography can help determine whether more tests are needed and if there are other lesions too small to be felt in the same or the other breast. All suspicious lumps should be biopsied for a firm diagnosis.

Survival When Not Detected Early

If the cancer has spread to neighboring areas, the 5-year survival rate is 76%. For cancer that has spread to distant organs, the outcome is poor, with a 5-year survival rate of only 21%. Survival after diagnosis continues to decline beyond 5 years. About 67% of women survive 10 years, and 56% survive 15 years.

Early Detection Tip

The 5-year relative survival rate for localized breast cancer has increased from 72% in the 1940s to 97% today. This emphasizes the importance of regular mammograms and breast self-exams to catch the disease early.

Breast Self-Exam

Women should perform a breast self-exam (BSE) once a month. This exam requires more skill than a skin self-exam (detailed later), so you might wish to have a clinician coach you on how to do a proper BSE. Menstruating women should do a BSE two or three days after the period ends, when the breasts are least likely to be tender or swollen. Here is an effective seven-step method for BSE:[2]

Secondary prevention means using self-examination and screening tests to detect already-forming cancers at an early stage, before they produce obvious symptoms and when there is a good possibility the cancer can be stopped.

1. Stand before a mirror and inspect both breasts. Look for anything unusual, such as nipple discharge or skin puckering, dimpling, or scaling. Notice the normal size and

shape of each breast and the normal position of the nipple. Once you become familiar with your breasts, it will be easier to notice anything suspicious.

2. Clasp your hands behind your head and press them forward. Look in the mirror at the shape and contour of your breasts. Look for any changes in size and shape or any swelling, dimpling, rash, discoloration, or other unusual changes of the skin.

3. Press your hands firmly on your hips and bow slightly toward your mirror as you pull your shoulders and elbows forward. Look for any change in the shape or contour of your breasts.

4. It may be easier to do this step in the bath or shower, since the fingers glide over soapy skin, allowing you to concentrate on the texture underneath. Raise your left arm. Use three or four fingers of your right hand to probe your left breast firmly, carefully, and thoroughly. Keep your fingers flat and close together. Use enough pressure to feel deep into the breast, but not enough to dull sensation. Technique improves with a little practice.

Beginning at the outer edge, press the flat part of your fingers in small circles, moving the circles slowly around the breast. Work gradually toward the nipple. Be sure to cover the entire breast. Pay special attention to the area between breast and armpit, and include the armpit itself. Feel for any unusual lump or mass under the skin. A lump is unusual if you have not felt it during prior exams and it now stands out against the normal feel of your breast.

5. Gently squeeze the nipple and look for a discharge. If present, see your doctor (if you have a discharge at any time, have it checked). Repeat steps 4 and 5 on your right breast.

6. Repeat steps 4 and 5 lying down. Lie flat on your back, left arm over your head and a pillow or folded towel under your left shoulder. This position flattens the breast

and makes it easier to examine. Use the same circular motion described earlier. Repeat on your right breast. If your breasts are large, you may need to hold the side of each one steady, either with your other hand or by resting it against a wall.

7. If you feel something in one breast that appears unusual or different from before, check to see if it is present in your other breast. If it is, chances are good that your breasts are normal. A lump found a few days before or during your menstrual period calls for a reexamination when your period ends. A lump found at this time may often be due to the normal collection of fluid during your period. If the lump does not disappear before your next period, check with your doctor.

Prostate Cancer

Symptoms of prostate cancer include weak or halting urine flow; inability to urinate; difficulty starting or stopping the urine flow; frequent urination, especially at night; blood in the urine; pain or burning on urination; continuing pain in lower back, pelvis, or upper thighs. Most of these symptoms are nonspecific and may indicate conditions other than cancer, such as prostate enlargement or infection.

Screening
The American Cancer Society's guidelines for early detection stress prostate-specific antigen (PSA) blood tests and digital rectal exams (DRE) of the prostate gland.

Survival When Not Detected Early
The general survival rate (all stages combined) has increased from 67 to 89% during the past 20 years. Survival rate at 10 years is 67%, and at 15 years is a poorer 50%.

Early Detection Tip

The 5-year survival rate for localized tumors is 100%, but only 58% of all prostate cancers are discovered at this early stage.

Colorectal Cancer

Warning signs of colorectal cancer include bleeding from the rectum, blood in the stool, or a change in bowel habits such as frequency or regularity.

Screening

Beginning at age 50, men and women should have one of the following: a yearly fecal occult blood test plus flexible sigmoidoscopy every 5 years, or colonoscopy every 10 years, or double contrast barium enema every 5 to 10 years. A digital rectal examination should be done at the same time as sigmoidoscopy, colonoscopy, or double contrast barium enema. These tests offer the best opportunity to detect colorectal cancer at an early stage and to prevent some cancers by detection and removal of polyps (benign growths that may turn into cancer).

Individuals should begin screening earlier and/or undergo screening more often if they have one or more of the colorectal cancer risk factors listed in chapter 2.

Survival When Not Detected Early

The 1- and 5-year general survival rates are 81% and 62%, respectively. If the cancer has spread to neighboring organs or lymph nodes, the 5-year survival rate is 64%. For cancers that have spread to distant organs, the 5-year rate is only 7%. Survival continues to decline beyond 5 years, and the 10-year general survival rate is 51%.

Early Detection Tip

When detected early, in the localized stage, the 5-year survival rate is 92%. Unfortunately, only 37% of colorectal cancers are discovered at this stage.

Cervical Cancer

Symptoms of cervical cancer include abnormal vaginal bleeding or spotting, and abnormal vaginal discharge. Late signs are pain and systemic symptoms.

Screening

The Pap test is a simple procedure that can be performed as part of a pelvic exam. A small sample of cells is swabbed from the cervix, transferred to a slide, and examined under a microscope. Women who have been sexually active or have reached age eighteen should have a Pap test and a pelvic exam every year. After three or more consecutive annual exams with normal findings, the Pap test may be performed less frequently at the physician's judgment.

Survival

Generally, 89% of cervical cancer patients survive 1 year after diagnosis, and 69% survive 5 years.

Early Detection Tip

The 5-year survival rate for localized cancers is 91%. Unfortunately, only 54% of Caucasians and 40% of African Americans are diagnosed at this early stage. There is room for much improvement in early detection of this cancer.

Endometrial (Uterine) Cancer

The symptoms of endometrial cancer (cancer of the uterus) include abnormal uterine bleeding or spotting. Pain and systemic symptoms are late manifestations of the disease.

Screening

The Pap test is rarely effective in detecting endometrial cancer. Women forty and over should have an annual pelvic exam. If you are at very high risk for this cancer, you should have an endometrial biopsy at menopause and periodically afterward as a screening test.

Survival When Not Detected at Early Stage

The general 1-year survival rate is 92%. If diagnosed after spreading to neighboring tissue, the rate is 66%. Survival rates for whites exceed those for blacks by at least 15% at every stage.

Early Detection Tip

The 5-year survival rate for early stage cancer is 96%.

Ovarian Cancer

Ovarian cancer is often "silent," showing no obvious signs or symptoms early on. The most common sign is enlargement of the abdomen, caused by fluid buildup. Abnormal vaginal bleeding is rare. In women over forty, vague gastrointestinal symptoms such as stomach discomfort, gas, or distention that persists and can't be explained by other causes should be evaluated.

Screening

Unfortunately, there is no adequate screening method for ovarian cancer. The Pap test rarely finds ovarian cancer. Periodic, thorough pelvic exams should be done. Transvaginal ultrasound and a tumor marker, CA125, may assist diagnosis, but are not recommended for routine screening.

Survival When Not Detected at Early Stage

The general 1-year survival rate is 76%, the 5-year survival rate for all stages, 46%. The 5-year survival rate is 55% for disease that has spread to neighboring areas and 25% for distant disease.

Early Detection Tip

For early stage disease, the survival rate is 93%. Unfortunately, only about 24% of all cases are detected at the localized stage.

Oral Cavity and Pharynx Cancer

Symptoms of oral cavity and pharynx cancer include a bleeding sore that does not heal; a lump or thickening; or a persisting red or white patch. Difficulty chewing, swallowing, or moving the tongue or jaws are often late symptoms.

Survival

Eighty-one percent of patients survive 1 year after diagnosis. For all stages combined, the 5-year survival rate is 53%, and the 10-year rate is 43%.

Early Detection Tip

Cancer can form anywhere in the oral cavity, including the lip, tongue, mouth, and throat. During regular checkups, dentists and physicians should be observant for abnormal tissue changes so that cancer can be detected at an early, curable stage.

Skin Cancer

A change in the size or color of a mole or other darkly pigmented growth or spot, or the spread of pigmentation beyond its border may be a sign of the skin cancer called malignant melanoma. Other skin cancers may show themselves as scaliness, oozing, bleeding, itchiness, tenderness, or pain in a fixed location, or a change in the appearance of a bump or nodule. A skin lesion that seems to heal and then reappears in the same place is a potential sign of a basal cell cancer.

Screening

Early detection is critical, because many skin cancers can spread to other parts of the body quickly. Watching for changes in skin growths and for new growths is the best way to find early skin cancer. Do a skin self-exam regularly (see the sidebar, Skin Self-Exam).

Melanoma. Melanomas often start as small, mole-like growths that increase in size and change color. A simple ABCD rule outlines the warning signals of melanoma. A is for asymmetry: Half of the mole does not match the other half. B is for border irregularity: The edges are ragged, notched, or blurred. C is for color: The pigmentation is not uniform or is intensely black. D is for a diameter greater than 6 millimeters (about $1/4$ inch; 1 inch = 25 millimeters). Any sudden or progressive increase in size is especially significant.

Squamous cell cancer. A red or white sore of almost any kind that doesn't heal in three weeks; a scaly or crusty patch; a small nodule that progresses into a wartlike lump.

Basal cell carcinoma. Any sore that changes in size or color; hurts, itches, or bleeds; any sore that doesn't heal in three weeks; a translucent, flesh-colored, pearly, or red nodule; a scaly, off-white or yellow patch resembling scar tissue; a blue, brown, or black lesion.[3]

Survival
The general 5-year survival rate for patients with malignant melanoma is 88%. The rate is 61% for disease confined to neighboring areas and 16% for distant disease. The survival rates of other types of skin cancer vary by type but are generally much better.

Early Detection Tip
When detected in its earliest stages, malignant melanoma, the most dangerous form of skin cancer, is highly curable. When localized, the 5-year relative survival rate is 95%. About 82% of melanomas are diagnosed at a localized stage. For basal cell or squamous cell cancers, cure is highly likely if detected and treated early.

Skin Self-Exam

Dermatologists recommend that you examine your skin periodically (for example, once a month) in front of a full-length mirror with good lighting. Use a hand mirror or have your partner examine your back, scalp, and other hard-to-see areas. Remember to look in between the toes and the bottom of the feet—anywhere there is skin. Once you become familiar with your skin, it will be easier to notice anything suspicious. See a doctor if you spot a new mole or growth that appears to be growing or changing. If you're over forty, it's prudent to see a dermatologist once a year for a head-to-toe professional exam. What are the benefits of a self-exam? Researchers at Sloan-Kettering and Yale interviewed 316 men over seven years, and found that men who examined their skin regularly lowered their melanoma risk 34%.[4]

Lung Cancer

The symptoms of lung cancer include a persistent cough, sputum (substance coughed up) streaked with blood, chest pain, and recurring pneumonia or bronchitis.

Screening

Because symptoms often do not appear until the disease is advanced, early detection is difficult. Chest x ray, analysis of cells contained in sputum, and fiber optic examination of the bronchial passages may help.

Survival

The 1-year survival rate has increased from 32% in 1973 to 40% in 1994, largely due to improvements in surgery. The 5-year survival rate for all stages combined is only 14%.

Table 3. Cure Rates for Localized Cancers (in %)

Cancer	% Cured
Prostate	100
Basal-cell carcinoma (skin)	99
Squamous-cell carcinoma (skin)	95
Melanoma (skin)	95
Breast (female)	97
Endometrial (uterine)	96
Ovarian	93
Colorectal	92
Cervical	91
Lung	49

Early Detection Tip

The early detection of lung cancer does not provide as promising an outcome as for other cancers. The survival rate is 49% for cases detected when the disease is still localized, but only 15% of lung cancers are discovered that early.

This emphasizes the importance of quitting or never starting to smoke, the major risk factor. There is a ray of light: In those who stop smoking when precancerous changes are found, damaged lung tissue often returns to normal.

Most major cancers, with the exception of lung cancer, have remarkably successful cure rates when detected and treated early. (For a quick recap of the cure rates for cancers detected and treated at an early stage, see table 3.)

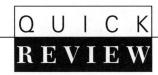

- Detecting and treating cancer early greatly increases the likelihood of a cure. The 5-year relative survival rate (cure rate) for screening-accessible cancers is about 80%. Regular screenings could increase that success rate to over 95%.

- Screenings for colon, cervical, and breast cancer have saved countless lives. Genetic screening for high-risk individuals will expand as more cancer-predisposing genes are identified. In addition to screening tests conducted by a health-care professional, you should regularly perform self-exams for breast and skin cancer.

- The mnemonic term CAUTION helps you remember cancer's seven general warning symptoms:

    Change in bowel or bladder habits.

    A sore that doesn't heal.

    Unusual bleeding or discharge.

    Thickening or lump in breast or elsewhere.

    Indigestion or difficulty in swallowing.

    Obvious change in wart or mole.

    Nagging cough or hoarseness.

Eat an Anticancer Diet

T hese next three chapters are the heart of the book:
foods and nutritional supplements that help you
reduce your cancer risk. Here you will find the essential information you need to actively protect yourself
and your family.

Foods Versus Supplements:
What's the Difference?

Chemopreventive agents are chemicals or compounds that
have a preventive effect against cancer. They can be synthetic drugs, vitamins or minerals in supplement form, or
bioactive compounds called *phytochemicals* (*phyto* is
from the Greek word for plant) present naturally in foods
and herbs.

Most evidence showing the cancer-preventive effects
of nutrients and phytochemicals in humans has come
from studies involving foods, not supplements. Singling
out a nutrient and putting it into a supplement may *not* be

the same as getting it from food in the diet. For example, studies show that foods high in beta-carotene appear to *lower* lung cancer risk in people who smoke, while beta-carotene supplements appear to *increase* the risk. (We'll look more closely at possible reasons for this apparent paradox later.) Foods contain thousands of substances, and currently no one knows exactly which ones work together or how they work together. Without supporting studies, there's no assurance that a particular nutrient in supplement form will have the same cancer-preventive effects shown by foods containing that nutrient.

However, some nutrients, including vitamin E and selenium, have been found to reduce cancer risk when taken as concentrated supplements. Numerous studies are underway to refine our knowledge about how well supplemental nutrients work.

Foods and nutritional supplements can help you reduce your cancer risk.

It seems reasonable to think that certain nutritional supplements can confer some protection against cancer, but they cannot make up for inattention to other aspects of a healthful lifestyle, such as diet, exercise, not smoking, and being moderate in drinking alcoholic beverages. As Jeffrey Blumberg, Ph.D., chief of the antioxidants research lab at the USDA Human Nutrition Research Center on Aging at Tufts University in Boston put it, taking a nutritional supplement is "like wearing a seatbelt—it gives you a measure of protection, but it does not give you a license to drive recklessly." In other words, don't be lulled into a false sense of security and think that taking nutritional supplements is all you need to do.

The synergistic approach is the one to aim for: Eat an anticancer diet *and* take nutritional supplements shown to have anticancer effects. One day it might be possible to identify key nutrients and phytochemicals and cobble them together into a pill that will ward off cancer regardless of the foods you eat. Until then, your best bet is to use a combination of diet and supplements.

Sometimes you will see the term *chemoprevention* used in a stricter sense to refer to agents in supplement form only and not to whole foods. The line is blurring, though, as the dietary supplement industry responds to intense consumer interest. Supplements are now available that provide not only traditional vitamins and minerals, but herbs and even whole-food concentrates such as cruciferous vegetables (broccoli, cabbage, cauliflower, and others) in extract or freeze-dried form. Not enough is known yet whether these whole-food formulations work as well as nature's versions, but they might come nearer to providing the protection of whole foods than single-nutrient supplements. They might be a reasonable alternative for people who, for whatever reason, cannot eat a balanced diet the traditional way.

Singling out a nutrient and putting it into a supplement is not the same as getting it from food in the diet.

This chapter covers *whole* foods—foods to avoid or cut back on (dietary fats, red meats, foods prepared or preserved certain ways), and foods to eat (fruits and vegetables, whole grains, legumes). Chapters 5 and 6 cover the *parts* of the whole— the bioactive components of whole foods that may possess anticancer effects, most of which are available in supplement form.

Benefits of a Plant-Rich Diet

"Up until 200 years ago, 80% of our diet came from plant products," said Oliver Alabaster of the Institute for Disease Prevention, George Washington University Medical Center. "That has now decreased to less than 50%, and because our bodies are not genetically adapted to that change, we are experiencing an epidemic of cancer and heart disease that is potentially avoidable."[1]

When life on earth began, plants lived in an environment without oxygen. Along the course of evolution, they began the process of taking in carbon dioxide and giving off oxygen, and, in so doing, polluted the environment with unstable forms of oxygen (free radicals). The plants learned to manufacture phytochemicals as part of their antioxidant defense system. The chemicals also served to protect them from viral and fungal attack, sunlight, and harsh weather. Living organisms—including humans—that fed on these plants apparently evolved to use these plant protectants the same way.

"There's an explosion of compelling and consistent data associating diets rich in fruits and vegetables with a lower cancer risk," said epidemiologist Tim Byers.

When you comb through the study data, it seems that the most *certain* cancer-preventive insurance you can find is eating the right foods. "There's an explosion of compelling and consistent data associating diets rich in fruits and vegetables with a lower cancer risk," said epidemiologist Tim Byers of the Centers for Disease Control and

Prevention in Atlanta, Georgia. At least 200 population studies worldwide have confirmed the link between a plant-rich diet and lower risk for several types of cancers. The key to this impressive protection may be that many of the hundreds of phytochemicals in nature's finely tuned botanical orchestra work together against cancer. A single ingredient, taken out of its natural context, may lose its powers.

It's estimated that 30%—and perhaps up to 70%—of all cases of cancer are linked to what we eat. The National Cancer Institute (a government organization) and the American Cancer Society (a private organization) and other groups have acknowledged the connection between diet and cancer and have issued dietary guidelines to help people reduce their risk.

Many people associate the word *diet* with eating to lose weight, as in a "crash diet" or some other temporary diet method touting the weight-reducing benefits of certain foods. Here, the word refers to eating a variety of foods in the "balanced diet" sense, and is intended to be a permanent fixture of a healthful lifestyle. Eating a balanced diet of enjoyable foods that can reduce your cancer risks and at the same time improve your overall health does not require as much effort as you might think. According to surveys, about one-third of Americans have already modified their diets for health reasons, and you can do it too.[2]

It's estimated that 30 to 70% of all cases of cancer are linked to what we eat.

Cancer is unique in that it is a disease involving the growth and replication of living cells. The problem is that the process has jerked out of control. Some researchers think that a poor diet may play a role primarily in the promotion stage of cancer, and others think diet may interact with all stages of cancer. You may recall the two-hit theory mentioned in chapter 1: *Initiation* is a quick, permanent hit, while *promotion* is a slower, progressive process that can stretch over years. Let's consider an example. A cell damaged by an initiator such as a mutation or a cancer-causing chemical passes on its abnormal genetic material to new cells. The potential for cancer is there, but a promoter is required for its eventual development. Over time, a diet high in fats, along with the effect of hormones, could promote tumor growth.

It's likely that many people carry around these damaged precancer cells, which wait stealthily to grow and spread without restraint. Because it takes a long time for most premalignant lesions to invade surrounding tissue and spread, promotion may be reversible in its early stages. This presents an important window of opportunity in which dietary and nutritional changes can help prevent cancer.

Foods to Avoid or Reduce

Some foods and agents are associated with an increased risk of cancer, and avoiding them or reducing your consumption of them is a key way to protect yourself against the disease. Discussed in this section are fats, red meat, meats cooked in certain ways, aflatoxins, pesticides, and food additives.

Fats

Fats are found in both animal and plant sources. Fat is a type of lipid, which also includes oils, waxes, and related compounds that do not mix with water. The terms *fats* and *fatty acids* are often used interchangeably. The three types of fats are saturated, polyunsaturated, and monounsaturated. Fats actually consist of a mixture of the three types and are categorized according to which type is predominant:

- *Saturated fats* include animal fats (beef, pork, and lamb), butter, cream, cream cheese, mayonnaise, salad dressings, coconut and palm oils, and most shortenings (hydrogenated oils).
- *Polyunsaturated fats* include most margarines, vegetable oils (corn, safflower, sunflower, soybean, sesame, and flaxseed), and seeds (flaxseed, sesame, sunflower, and pumpkin).
- *Monounsaturated fats* include olive oil (by far the most monounsaturated of the monounsaturated fats), canola oil, peanut oil, avocado oil, and some margarines.[3]

Fat and Cancer

The association between dietary fat and heart disease has been extensively studied and leaves little doubt that

Though smoking poses the single greatest risk for lung cancer, studies have suggested that dietary fat may also be a contributing factor.

diets high in saturated fats (from animal sources) and trans-fatty acids (found in margarine and other hydrogenated foods) increase LDL cholesterol levels, and in turn, the risk of heart disease.[4] However, the connection between dietary fats and cancer is still under debate. Most researchers do believe that fat is associated with increased cancer risk—it's just that the types of clinical trials needed for conclusive proof have not been done. The current evidence relies primarily on laboratory or animal results[5] as well as observational studies demonstrating associations between dietary fat intake and cancers of the breast, prostate, and colon.[6] In the latter, it is difficult to isolate the effects of fats from that of other dietary components.

Fat is thought to be a direct or indirect cancer promoter, speeding up the cancer process in abnormal cells. In breast cancer, for instance, fat may coax the body to produce more estrogen, which can promote cancer. Similarly, excess fat is believed to play a role in prostate cancer in men. Fat may also increase cancer risk through oxidative breakdown products formed when it turns rancid, a process that unleashes damaging free radicals.

To test the hypothesis that dietary fat may contribute to the development of hormone-related cancers such as ovarian cancer, researchers interviewed 450 women ages 35 to 79 concerning reproduction and diet, as well as 564 randomly selected population control subjects. They found that saturated fat consumption was associated with a 20% increased risk of ovarian cancer for each 10 g of daily intake. No such link was found for unsaturated fats.[7]

Though smoking poses the single greatest risk for lung cancer, studies have suggested that dietary fat may also be a contributing factor. In one study, a food frequency questionnaire was used to obtain dietary information on 429 female nonsmoking white women ages 30 to 84 who had a

There's quite a bit of suggestive evidence that a high-fat diet promotes the development of postmenopausal breast cancer, but we don't yet have conclusive evidence.

diagnosis of lung cancer, as well as 1,021 control subjects.[8] The women were interviewed before any cancer might have changed eating patterns. Researchers found that those who ate the most saturated fat had more than a sixfold greater risk of developing lung cancer than those who ate the least. This rate was higher than expected, based on earlier studies. Additionally, the effect of saturated fat was more pronounced for a cancer called adenocarcinoma than for other cell types.

This does not conclusively prove that dietary fat increases lung cancer risk. As some researchers point out, fat could serve merely as a marker for some other risk, such as carcinogenic substances (heterocyclic amines) that form when red meat is cooked.

There's quite a bit of suggestive evidence that a high-fat diet promotes the development of postmenopausal breast cancer. The evidence comes from various sources: data showing high correlations between fat intake and breast cancer rates, links between a high-fat diet and breast cancer in case-control studies, and animal model studies consistently demonstrating that dietary fat influences breast cancer development at several stages in the carcinogenic process.

Studies suggest that consumption of saturated fat increases the risk of prostate and colorectal cancer.

However, large prospective studies have found little evidence that saturated fats increase the risk of breast cancer. Studies do suggest that consumption of saturated fat increases the risk of prostate cancer;[9] and research evidence indicates that an increased intake of fat and red meat is associated with a higher risk of colorectal cancer, probably prostate cancer, and possibly breast and other cancers.[10] Conclusive evidence can come only from intervention trials which have not yet been performed.[11]

How to Cut Fat from Your Diet

Overall fat intake should not exceed 30% of daily calories from the diet. Some experts think that's too much, and that 20% would be better. Before the new Nutrition Facts food label came about (see figure 1 and discussion later), you had to look up foods in a reference guide and make calculations to determine the number of fat calories and grams you were getting. The Nutrition Facts food label appears on packaged foods and does this for you, so it's easier than ever before to be aware of what you're doing.

Here are a few key ways to cut significant amounts of fat from your diet:

- Become familiar with the Nutrition Facts food label and consult it when purchasing foods.
- Eat less red meat—substitute chicken and fish instead.
- Pick lean meats and chicken. Remove the skin from chicken before cooking or eating. Trim away visible fat before eating.
- Use less butter, margarine, and oils (cooking oils, salad dressings, and so on). Use olive oil for cooking and salad dressings. Cut out or use less mayonnaise or similar dressings on sandwiches.
- Choose lowfat or skim-milk dairy products instead of whole milk and cream.
- Broil, roast, or poach meats and drain off fat after cooking.

However, certain forms of fat, such as that found in olive oil, may actually be good for you. More on this later.

Red Meat

Red meat—beef, pork, and lamb—has been linked to several cancers, particularly colon and prostate cancer, and

possibly breast and pancreatic cancer. Harvard researcher Edward Giovannucci's 1993 study of 51,529 men found a 2.64 times greater risk of prostate cancer in the high red meat consumption group compared to those in the low red meat consumption group.[12]

> **Red meat—beef, pork, and lamb— has been linked to several cancers.**

Harvard researcher Walter Willett's 1990 study of 88,751 women found that those who ate the most red meat and the least chicken and fish were 2.49 times as likely to get colon cancer as those at the opposite extreme.[13]

The apparent increased cancer risk could be due to the high saturated fat content of meat rather than an inherent component of meat. However, some forms of meat may directly increase cancer risk.

Dangerous By-Products from Cooking Meats

Cooking meats at high temperatures (frying, grilling) and for a long duration produces heterocyclic amines (HCAs), known cancer-causing compounds. Additionally, barbecuing or grilling meats produces polycyclic aromatic hydrocarbons (PAHs). Frequent eating of grilled or barbecued meats may increase the chances of getting cancer of the stomach or esophagus, according to a 1997 study.[14] Of cooking methods, grilling and barbecuing were associated with an increased cancer risk, while broiling or frying were not.

The study also looked at degree of doneness as a separate issue. A preference for eating beef cooked well-done—compared to rare or medium rare—was associated with a 3.2 times greater risk of stomach cancer, but not esophageal cancer. Medium and medium-well carried a 2.4 times greater risk.

There's some good news for outdoor grillers. A recent study demonstrated that marinating meats may dramatically reduce the amounts of carcinogens associated with grilling.[15] Researchers at the Lawrence Livermore National Laboratory in California cooked skinless, boneless chicken breast on a propane gas grill after marinating it in a brown sugar–cider vinegar mixture with oil, lemon juice, and spices. What was the result? The chicken had between 92% and 99% fewer of the potential carcinogens—heterocyclic aromatic amines—than unmarinated chicken. When the chicken was *overcooked* until it became dry, tough, or charred, it did contain more of a potent heterocyclic amine called MeIQx. And don't worry too much about the marinade fat content. "Even just briefly dipping the chicken into the marinade and then blotting it before grilling coats it enough to reduce the heterocyclic amines," said Mark Knize, one of the researchers.

Cooking meats at high temperatures (frying, grilling) and for a long duration produces cancer-causing compounds.

Here are some additional tips from the American Cancer Society:

- Use foil or a drop pan when grilling. When fat from the meats falls into the coals, chips, heating element, or flames, the smoke also produces carcinogens, which can land on the food.

- Choose lowfat cuts of meat. Trim away as much fat and skin as possible. Serve only 3- to 4-ounce portions. This will reduce fat intake and prevent the formation of carcinogens.
- Barbecue or grill to finish cooking meats to add special flavor. Precook by baking, boiling, or microwaving halfway through, lessening time on the grill and eliminating some fat.
- Skewer your meat because smaller pieces will reduce cooking time and fat intake.

Potential Problems with Grains, Nuts, and Seeds: Aflatoxins

Aflatoxins are potent carcinogens and immune system suppressants produced by a fungus. They can develop in grains, nuts, and seeds when they become moldy, which can happen when they are harvested or stored.[16] Studies have linked aflatoxins to liver and esophageal cancer in several countries where contaminated foods are commonplace. To protect yourself, keep these food items sealed and dry and discard any that have become moldy or damp.

Marinating meats may dramatically reduce the amounts of carcinogens associated with grilling.

Pesticides

The agricultural industry dumps tons of chemical pesticides on crops to control pest infestations, and some of the residue remains on many of our foods. The potential cancer-causing effects of pesticides have long been debated. Some experts say the effect is nil, and point out that naturally occurring pesticides—which evolved to ward off attacks by natural pests—are more prevalent in the foods we eat than are manufactured pesticides.

Animal studies using doses far exceeding what is normally consumed do link some pesticides and food additives to cancer. However, a panel of international experts convened by the American Institute for Cancer Research (AICR) and the World Cancer Research Fund recently reviewed diet and cancer findings from over 4,500 studies. They found no convincing evidence that food additives or pesticide residues were harmful to humans when consumed in the amounts typically found in foods.[17] Without the use of pesticides and herbicides, the quantity and quality of fruits and vegetables making it to market might significantly decline.

Still, it seems prudent to keep your intakes of these "iffy" compounds as low as practically possible. One way to do that is to use organically grown natural produce, cultivated without pesticides. Aside from that, it's a good idea to thoroughly wash all fruits and vegetables before eating to remove as much pesticide residue as possible. Be aware that soaking produce can draw out nutrients. Remove outer leaves of leafy vegetables such as lettuce and cabbage, since they are likely to carry the highest level of contaminants. If possible, buy American-grown produce, because that grown in foreign countries may be treated with more dangerous pesticides banned or restricted in the United States.

Carcinogens can develop in grains, nuts, rice, and seeds when they become moldy. Keep these food items sealed and dry.

Food Additives

The controversy over food additives is as big a jumble as that over pesticides, with much squabbling among federal regulatory agencies, environmental activist groups, and private industry. Food additives are chemical substances added to food to preserve freshness, improve taste, add color or thickness, and retain nutrient value.

Nitrites, typically sodium nitrite, are used as preservatives to maintain color and prevent bacterial contamination in meats such as bacon, ham, sausage, hot dog franks, and luncheon meats. Nitrites are also found in smoked and salt-pickled foods, and some baked products. In the stomach, nitrites combine with amines to form nitrosamines, carcinogenic compounds thought to be a major cause of cancer of the stomach and esophagus. Vitamin C and other antioxidants are often added to foods to help block this conversion.

There is no convincing evidence that pesticide residues are harmful to humans when consumed in the amounts typically found in foods.

Besides nitrites, *nitrates* are added to foods and also occur naturally in many vegetables. Nitrates can be converted into nitrites by digestive tract bacteria or by saliva. Nature apparently counterbalances the potential damage from nitrates by providing natural protectants such as vitamin C in the same vegetables. Taking supplemental antioxidants may provide extra protection from nitrites added to processed foods. The American Cancer Society, however, does not regard nitrates as a significant cause of cancer among Americans.

There are dozens of other additives in foods. The law called the Delaney clause, enacted in response to the cancer scare of the 1950s, was designed to protect Americans from exposure to carcinogens by banning all cancer-causing agents. In effect, the law specified a zero-tolerance approach to potential carcinogens in food, without regard to the dose or level of a potential carcinogen.[18] For example, if a

Supplemental antioxidants may provide extra protection from nitrites added to processed foods.

substance causes cancer in lab animals when given at extremely high doses, it is regarded as unsafe in any amount for human consumption. Critics argue that it is time to change this approach to regulating food additives. According to the American Cancer Society, food additives are usually present in very small quantities, and there is no convincing evidence that any additive at these levels causes human cancers.

You can't wash away additives, so if you want additive-free foods, your only option is to use organically grown natural produce. Again, taking nutritional supplements may provide extra protection.

It may offer some comfort to know that two of the most commonly used antioxidant food preservatives, BHA and BHT, may have a cancer-*preventive* effect in humans.[19] Dr. Andrew Dannenberg, of Cornell Medical College, found that these compounds "revved up" the gene that produces an enzyme that helps destroy carcinogens. The preservatives appear to work in a similar way to the phytochemical sulforaphane in broccoli and other plants. Both activate the same gene.

The Other Side of the Issue: Foods You Should Eat

Just as avoiding certain foods can reduce your cancer risk, so can making sure you eat certain foods. The best evidence is for fruits and vegetables.

Eat Your Vegetables!

Diet and cancer studies show that you can significantly reduce your cancer risk if you eat a diet high in plant foods (fruits, vegetables, grains, and beans). Eating lots of fruits and vegetables lowers the risk of several cancers, including lung, oral, pancreas, larynx, esophagus, bladder, and stomach. The data is not as strong for hormone-related cancers of the prostate, breast, ovary, and endometrium.[20]

You can significantly reduce your cancer risk if you eat a diet high in plant foods.

The benefit of a high plant food diet appears to be a general one that is consistently found with many different groups of fruits and vegetables. A diet emphasizing plant foods provides your body with protective vitamins, minerals, and phytochemicals. Eating this way can make a big impact on the 30% or more cancers related to a poor diet.

Monounsaturated Fats and Breast Cancer

Though excessive overall fat intake is thought to increase the risk of cancer, a recent study suggests that monounsaturated fats may actually have a protective effect. This type of fat is found in high concentrations in olive oil and canola oil. Researchers at the Karolinska Institute in Stockholm, Sweden, followed 61,471 women aged 40 to 76 years who had no previous diagnosis of cancer.[21]

The women who consumed the most monounsaturated fats had a 20% lower risk of breast cancer. This also confirmed previous studies showing that olive oil reduced breast cancer rates.[22] The study authors noted that the entire group of monounsaturated fats, not just olive oil, appeared to be beneficial, going so far as to say, "Research investigations and health policy considerations should take into account the emerging evidence that monounsaturated fat might be protective for risk of breast cancer."

Like monounsaturated fats, polyunsaturated fats are believed to be a healthy substitute for saturated fats in the diet. We know that both types significantly lower cholesterol levels. However, polyunsaturated fats have not been associated with any protective effect against cancer. One explanation may be that monounsaturated fats are less prone to oxidize and conjure up damaging free radicals, which may play a role in cancer development.

The women who consumed the most monounsaturated fats (for example, olive oil and canola oil) had a 20% lower risk of breast cancer.

Another advantage of monounsaturated oils is that highly polyunsaturated oils don't hold up well to heat. Heating them speeds oxidation and the production of free radicals. In any case, once heated, oils should not be reused, because that can induce further oxidation. The best oils for cooking are thought to be olive oil and canola oil, composed mainly of oleic acid, a monounsaturated oil more resistant to heat and light than highly polyunsaturated oils. Extra-virgin and virgin olive oil are the highest quality, made from first pressing the olives without added chemicals, but less expensive olive oils may still be healthy for you. Peanut oil may be a good choice for deep frying, and olive oil can be used in sautéing in place of butter or margarine.

Fiber: What You Can't Digest Can Be Good for You

Fiber, sometimes called roughage, creates bulk in the intestines, and may also help prevent cancer. The National Cancer Institute recommends 25 to 35 g of dietary fiber a day, but most Americans get only about 10 g. This may be the reason that the Chinese, who consume much higher levels of fiber, have a lower incidence of colon cancer and heart disease than Americans.

Heating polyunsaturated oils speeds oxidation and the production of free radicals.

Fiber is found only in plant foods like whole-grain breads and cereals, beans and peas, and other vegetables and fruits. It is the indigestible structural part of plants such as celery strings, corn-kernel skins, the membrane sections of an orange, and the bran that surrounds grains. The two types of fiber are soluble and insoluble. Soluble fiber can lower blood cholesterol, and includes that found in oat bran, rice bran, barley, guar gum, pectin, and cooked dried beans. Insoluble fiber appears to provide the best protection against colon cancer, and includes that found in wheat bran and the woody parts of fruits and vegetables.[23]

However, this issue is not settled. The surprising results of a recent analysis from the huge Harvard Nurses' Health Study found no evidence that eating more high-fiber foods lowered the risk of colon cancer.[24] This was an observational study, so it may be open to at least some question. For example, an earlier analysis from the same study found no evidence that fiber had a preventive effect against breast cancer, while several other studies did find a fiber-protective effect. The problem is that it's hard to tell whether it's the fiber or other components of fruits and vegetables exerting the benefit. Also, diets high in fiber tend to be low in fat, so it could be that getting less fat is what's important. Studies continue to evaluate the benefits of fiber in cancer prevention. There is little doubt that fiber helps protect against heart disease.

Whole-grain breads, cereals, pasta, and rice are high in fiber and low in fat. Vegetables and fruits are also good sources of fiber. High-fiber vegetables, starting with the highest fiber content, include acorn squash, black beans, artichokes, lima beans, chickpeas, great northern beans, kidney beans, potatoes (with skin), yams, and peas. High-fiber fruits, starting with the highest fiber content, include avocados, raspberries, black-berries, seedless raisins, apples, figs, guavas, pears, blueberries, and mangoes.[25] To get different types of fiber, you need to eat a variety of fruits and vegetables, so don't limit your selections to just one or two favorites. An-

Fiber may also help prevent cancer.

other reason for variety is that different fruits and vegetables contain different nutrients and you need them all.

Tip: Because fiber is indigestible, you may experience bloating, gas, and intestinal discomfort if you eat too much too quickly. So increase your fiber foods slowly over a period of time to give your body a chance to adjust.

The Nutrition Facts Food Label: Help at the Grocery Store

The United States Department of Agriculture's Nutrition Facts food label is a boon for health-conscious consumers

High-fiber fruits include avocados, raspberries, blackberries, seedless raisins, apples, figs, guavas, pears, blueberries, and mangoes.

(see figure 1). The label enables you to select health-smart foods that will help ward off cancer and other diseases such as heart disease. It's required on most packaged foods, but not on certain ready-to-eat foods like unpackaged deli and bakery items and restaurant food. Labels are also voluntary for many raw foods, such as fish, meat, poultry, and raw fruits and vegetables that are most frequently consumed.

Once you familiarize yourself with it, the label is easy to use. All manufacturers are required to use the same label format clearly stating the serving size (in both household and metric measures), number of servings per container, and the number of calories per serving. But that's just the beginning.

The label in figure 1 details the nutrition facts for a package of cookies. The bold line across the middle divides it into two parts. The top part presents information about an individual serving of that product. The first line states that one serving size (three cookies) contains 180 calories, 90 of which are calories from fat. Next comes key information on the food components most associated with maintaining good health—fat (total and saturated), cholesterol, sodium, carbohydrates (including fiber and sugars), and protein.

Look at fat content, for example. An individual serving provides 10 g of total fat, which is 15% of the recommended total daily value (amount). Most dietary guidelines recommend that you get no more than 30% of total daily

Nutrition Facts

Serving Size 3 cookies (34g/1.2 oz)
Servings Per Container About 5

Amount Per Serving

Calories 180	Calories from Fat 90

	%Daily Value*
Total Fat 10g	**15%**
Saturated Fat 3.5g	**18%**
Polyunsaturated Fat 1g	
Monounsaturated Fat 5g	
Cholesterol 10mg	**3%**
Sodium 80g	**3%**
Total Carbohydrate 21g	**7%**
Dietary Fiber 1g	**4%**
Sugars 11g	
Protein 2g	

Vitamin A 0%	•	Vitamin C 0%
Calcium 0%	•	Iron 4%
Thiamin 6%	•	Riboflavin 4%
Niacin 4%		

*Percent Daily Values are based on a 2,000 calorie diet. Your daily values may be higher or lower depending on your calorie needs:

	Calories	2,000	2,500
Total Fat	Less than	65g	80g
Sat Fat	Less than	20g	25g
Cholesterol	Less than	300mg	300mg
Sodium	Less than	2,400mg	2,400mg
Total Carbohydrate		300g	375g
Dietary Fiber		25g	30g

Ingredients: Unbleached enriched wheat flour (flour, niacin, reduced iron, thiamin mononitrate [vitamin B₁]), sweet chocolate (sugar, chocolate liquor, cocoa butter, soy lecithin added as an emulsifier, vanilla extract), sugar, partially hydrogenated vegetable shortening (soybean, cottonseed and/or canola oils), nonfat milk, whole eggs, cornstarch, egg whites, salt, vanilla extract, baking soda, and soy lecithin.

Serving Size reflects the amount typically eaten by many people.

The list of nutrients covers those most important to the health of today's consumers.

Calories from Fat are now shown on the label to help consumers meet dietary guidelines that recommend people get no more than 30 percent of the calories in their overall diet from fat.

% Daily Value (DV) shows how a food in the specified serving size fits into the overall daily diet. By using the % DV you can easily determine whether a food contributes a lot or a little of a particular nutrient. And you can compare different foods with no need to do any calculations.

Figure 1. *The Nutrition Facts Food Label*

calories from fat. (The math is done for you. The label is standardized to a 2,000-calorie diet, and 30% of 2,000 calories is 600 calories. Each gram of fat has 9 calories, so 600 divided by 9 is approximately 65 g. Ten grams, the amount of fat in a serving of this product, is 15% of 65 grams.)

Shift your attention to the lower half of the label, below the information on vitamins, and you'll see columns in smaller print. This is the reference section, and the numbers it shows are the same on all food labels—it's there as a reminder for you. These numbers are the total daily values (amounts) associated with a 2,000-calorie diet and a 2,500-calorie diet. The 2,000 column shows 65 g of total fat. Though information is listed for a 2,500-calorie diet, the individual serving information in the top half of the label is based on a 2,000-calorie diet. If you are on a diet with fewer than 2,000 calories or more than 2,500 calories, you may have to do a bit of figuring yourself. However, once you become accustomed to the label, you will be able to estimate fairly closely for other caloric amounts.

The last item at the bottom of the label tells you the number of calories per gram of fat (9), carbohydrates (4), and protein (4). As you can see, fat is the highest source of dietary calories. The bottom line: If you eat those three cookies, you've consumed 15% of the recommended allotted fat intake for the day (if you're on a 2,000-calorie diet). The fat can add up fast.

A tip: The USDA has determined that the average person eats about 20 food items a day. To stay on target, your fat intake should average 5% per food item ($5\% \times 20 = 100\%$), though you'll go above or below the average on individual products. Some experts think that the 30% target is too high and recommend getting less than 20% of calories from fat. The new food label is a giant step forward in helping you control your fat intake as well as increase your fiber intake and be savvy about other aspects of your diet.

The Food Guide Pyramid Is Your Map to Healthful Eating

The food guide pyramid is another useful tool devised by the USDA (see figure 2). It replaces the prior Basic Four Food Groups and divides foods into six groups with a recommended number of daily servings from each group. One of its purposes is to steer Americans away from diets high in fat toward nutritionally balanced meals that contain more complex carbohydrates (starch and fiber).

In the pyramid, the most important foods are those closest to the base and taking up the largest area in the illustration. The level one group consists of bread, cereal, pasta, and rice; level two consists of the vegetable and fruit groups; level three consists of the milk, yogurt, cheese group and the meat, poultry, fish, dry beans, eggs, nuts group; level four at the top consists of the fats, oils, and sweets group. Though dry beans (such as pinto, navy, kidney, and black beans) are included in the meat and beans group as meat alternatives, they can count as vegetables instead.

As you can see, you should choose most of your foods from the grain products group (6 to 11 servings), the vegetable group (3 to 5 servings), and the fruit group (2 to 4 servings). Most people need at least the minimum number of servings from each group daily. Eat moderate amounts from the milk group (2 to 3 servings) and the meat and beans group (2 to 3 servings). Eat sparing amounts from the fats and sweets group at the top—they provide few nutrients and may be high in fat and sugars (fats and sugars also occur naturally in the other food groups). The number of servings would vary according to the total calories in your diet. The smaller number of servings in each category is for people consuming about 1,600 calories a day and the larger number is for those consuming about 2,800 calories a day.

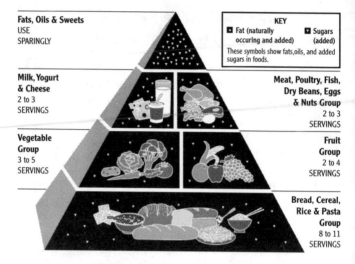

Figure 2. *The Food Guide Pyramid*

Besides the fats and oils group, you'll find high-fat foods in the milk–dairy group, meat–eggs–beans group, and in some processed foods in the bread–grains group. Use the Nutrition Facts food label to help you select foods low in fat, saturated fat, and cholesterol and higher in fiber. Saturated fat should make up less than 10% of calories (20 g per 2,000 calories) and dietary cholesterol should be held below 300 mg daily. It should be noted that children under age two need to consume a higher percentage of fat calories than adults.

The milk–dairy group provides most of the calcium in the American diet, in addition to vitamin D, conjugated linoleic acid, and other components that may lower cancer risk. To secure the benefits and bypass the fat hazard, choose skim or lowfat milk and nonfat yogurt.

Foods emphasized in the food guide pyramid—grains, fruits, and vegetables—are home to a wide array of vitamins, minerals, and phytochemicals that provide solid

protection against cancer and other chron
pected cancer-fighting phytochemicals and s
plant foods containing high levels of them includ
pene (tomatoes and pink grapefruit), isoflavone phyt
estrogens (soybean and soy products such as tofu and
non-dairy soy milk), polyphenol flavonoids (green tea),
organosulfides (garlic and onion), lignans (flaxseed), and
sulforaphane (Brassica or cruciferous vegetables such as
broccoli, kale, cauliflower, cabbage, brussels sprouts, and
mustard greens). These substances are discussed in detail
in the supplements chapters. Researchers are just scratch-
ing the surface, and fruits and vegetables may contain
hundreds of other yet unidentified potent phytochemicals.

Eating Right

Here are some key tips and guidelines to help you put
healthful, cancer-fighting foods on your dining table. Get
into the habit and, before long, you might even forget
your old way of eating.

Tips to Trim Dietary Fats

Here are some easy ways to cut down on the amount of fat
you eat:

- *Fats and Oils Group:* Use small amounts of salad
  dressings and spreads such as butter, margarine, and
  mayonnaise. Or use lowfat or fat-free dressings for
  salads or no dressings at all.
- *Bread–Grains, Vegetables, and Fruits Groups:* Eat
  lowfat sauces with pasta, rice, and potatoes. Use
  minimal fats and oils when cooking vegetables and
  grain products. For seasoning, use spices, herbs,
  lemon juice, and lowfat or fat-free salad dressings.
- *Meat–Eggs–Beans Group:* Select meats labeled
  "lean" or "extra lean." Trimming fat from meat and

ultry can cut fat by up to half.
t and good sources of fiber and
ar intake of processed meats and
eat these, use the Nutrition Facts
mpare fat grams. Limit organ meats
which tend to be high in cholesterol
o not contain cholesterol).

- *Milk* / *Group:* Use skim or lowfat milk, lowfat or fat-free yogurt, and lowfat cheese.

Tips on Cooking, Storing, and Preparing Foods

The cooking and storage methods you use can have a big impact on the nutrient value of the foods you eat. Here are some hints:

- The best cooking methods to preserve antioxidant nutrients are microwaving, steaming, and stir-frying.[26]
- Avoid cooking in water. Nutrients, especially the water-soluble C and B vitamins, tend to leach out into the water. Or consume the water you use in cooking.
- Avoid wilted produce. Store fresh vegetables in a refrigerator vegetable crisper or seal them in moisture-proof bags.
- Choose vegetables with the brightest or deepest colors. This generally indicates greater vitamin and phytamin content. For instance, romaine lettuce has several times more vitamin C than iceberg lettuce.
- Don't buy pre-cut produce. To keep nutrient levels at their peak, delay cutting and washing fruits and vegetables until just before cooking or eating them. Any exposure to light and heat can cause deterioration in nutrient content, especially antioxidants.
- Refrigerate once-cooked foods in air-tight containers and eat them within a day or two. Avoid storing

refrigerated fresh produce longer than a week, the sooner it's eaten, the better.

- Frozen fruits and vegetables may be a better choice if you think you won't eat fresh produce within a few days. "Vegetables are usually frozen within a few hours of harvest, so the nutritional quality can actually be better than fresh," said Diane Barrett, Ph.D., associate professor of food science and technology at the University of California at Davis. And frozen is better than canned.[27]

American Cancer Society Dietary Guidelines

To keep pace with the scientific evidence, the American Cancer Society issued new general nutrition guidelines in 1996 that are consistent with the USDA's food guide pyramid:

- Choose most of your foods from plant sources.
- Eat five or more servings of fruits and vegetables each day.
- Eat several servings from other plant sources (breads, cereals, grains, rice, pasta, beans) each day.
- Limit intake of high-fat foods, particularly from animal sources (saturated fat).
- Limit meats, especially high-fat meats.
- Be physically active; achieve and maintain a healthy weight.
- Be moderately active for 30 minutes or more on most days.
- Limit alcoholic beverages.

The 5-a-Day Challenge

The National Cancer Institute's 5-a-Day Challenge is designed to give you insight into your eating habits and help you and your family get started down the path to a healthful diet. The idea is to eat five servings of vegetables and fruits every day for a week. Here are the suggestions to help you get your five a day:

- Drink fruit or vegetable juice with breakfast.
- Have a piece of fresh fruit or raw vegetable sticks as a snack.
- Have a fruit salad or vegetable salad with lunch or dinner.
- Have a vegetable side dish with the main meal for the day.
- Have fresh fruit for dessert.
- Top your cereal with dried or fresh fruit.
- Add raw vegetables to your sandwich.
- Choose fruit-flavored, lowfat yogurt.
- Choose whole-grain breads with fruit.
- Add vegetables to other dishes.

When you use the Nutrition Facts food label and the food pyramid as guides to gradually introduce health-smart foods to your diet, you'll automatically be reducing your fat intake and increasing your fiber intake. Once you've made it a habit, there's no law saying you can't splurge now and then with a bag of fries or bowl of ice cream. The key is long-term consistency. Like many other people who have adapted to a balanced diet, you're apt to find yourself pleasantly surprised at how much better you feel and how much less of an attraction those high-fat treats have become.

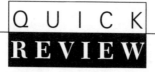

QUICK REVIEW

- **Thirty percent or more cancers are linked to the foods we eat. Over the generations, the move from a diet high in** plant-based foods to one significantly lower in plant foods may be one reason for higher rates of cancer.

- Vegetables, fruits, and whole grains contain essential vitamins and minerals as well as hundreds of phytochemicals that may protect against cancer and other chronic diseases such as heart disease.

  These natural compounds evolved to protect plants from free radicals and other environmental enemies and may function similarly in humans.

  Over 200 studies worldwide clearly show that a plant-rich diet lowers the risk for numerous cancers. The key to this protection may be the way nutrients and phytochemicals in foods work together against cancer.

  You can significantly lower your cancer risk by regularly eating certain foods and avoiding others.

- Avoid or reduce your consumption of fats (especially animal fats), red meat (beef, pork, and lamb), grilled or overcooked meats, pickled and salt-cured meats, and those in which aflatoxins are present.

- The evidence against food additives and pesticides is not strong—most experts think there's no convincing evidence that these substances are harmful when consumed in amounts typically found in foods. However, an option is to eat organically grown produce.

- Evidence suggests that a diet high in fats may be linked to an increased risk of several cancers, including those of the breast, ovary, prostate, colon, and lung. Red meats are linked to an increased risk of colon and prostate cancer, and possibly breast and pancreatic cancer. Polyunsaturated or monounsaturated fats should be substituted for saturated fats in the diet. Monounsaturated fats may offer some advantages. For example, they are less likely to produce free radicals than polyunsaturated fats. Additionally, mono-unsaturated fats such as olive oil may actually have a protective effect against breast cancer and possibly other cancers.

- Emphasizing foods low in fat and high in fiber can significantly reduce your risk of cancer. The USDA's Nutrition Facts food label and food guide pyramid are valuable tools that make it easier than ever before to select health-smart foods. See the text for tips on how to cut down on dietary fats and the best ways to prepare and store foods, as well as nutrition tips and guidelines from the American Cancer Society and the National Cancer Institute.

Vitamins and Minerals That May Reduce Your Cancer Risk

T he nutrients we need to sustain life comprise six categories: proteins, carbohydrates, fats, vitamins, minerals, and water. Proteins, carbohydrates, and fats furnish calories and provide our bodies with energy. Vitamins and minerals are vital in the regulation of all body processes, but do not provide calories or energy. Water is essential to support all body processes.

Vitamins

Vitamins are organic substances produced by living matter (animals and plants), while minerals are inorganic substances originating in soil. The 13 vitamins are called "essential" nutrients because the body cannot make them in adequate amounts—we must obtain them from what we eat. Similarly, 15 to 20 minerals and 1 oil (linoleic acid) are also considered essential nutrients.

Vitamins are broadly categorized as water-soluble and fat-soluble. The water-soluble vitamins—vitamin C and the B vitamins—are stored in the body only temporarily before they are washed out, and, as a consequence, frequent replenishment is necessary. The fat-soluble vitamins—A, D, E, and K—are readily stored by the body, which means that we can't run short of them easily, but at least some of them have the potential to build up and cause toxicity. The body can make vitamin A from another nutrient, beta-carotene.

Antioxidants

Vitamins A, beta-carotene, C, E, and the mineral selenium function as *antioxidants,* agents with the ability to deactivate toxic compounds called *free radicals.* Other substances in foods also have antioxidant activity, and the body produces its own antioxidants.

Oxygen-free radicals or oxidants are highly unstable molecules that can damage cell membranes and scramble the genetic information (DNA) in cells and start a chain reaction that may lead to cancer. They are produced in the body during normal cell metabolism, from tissue injury, and also as a result of exposure to tobacco smoke, sunlight, x rays, and other environmental sources.

Extensive evidence suggests that damage by free radicals is in part responsible for the development of cancer as well as other chronic diseases such as heart disease and diseases associated with aging. Researchers think

Free radicals are highly unstable molecules that can damage cell membranes, scramble the genetic information, and start a chain reaction that may lead to cancer.

that cancer cells themselves may generate a surplus of oxidants, which then send signals that promote uncontrolled cell growth, and that antioxidant nutrients may block the signals. "Control of signaling pathways involving oxidants may explain why some antioxidants appear to prevent development of certain cancers," said Keikobad Irani, M.D., of Johns Hopkins.[1]

Free radicals aren't entirely bad. For example, they help fend off disease by teaming up with the immune system to destroy bacteria and other foreign invaders. Problems occur when the production of free radicals overwhelms the body's ability to contain them. As with most things, balance is the key, and it is generally believed that a proper balance between free radicals and antioxidants is essential to good health. That's why the body's antioxidants try to gobble up excessive amounts of free radicals before they can cause damage.

> **The body's antioxidants try to gobble up excessive amounts of free radicals before they can cause damage.**

Understanding Research Studies

Because scientific research is the backbone of effective prevention and treatment of disease, the more you know about how these studies work the better your understanding will be. Before we continue, then, let's briefly define the types of studies.

Observational Study

An *observational* study (also called an *epidemiological* or *population* study) looks at large populations in an attempt to find trends. It is usually retrospective—that is, it examines what has happened in the past. Participants may fill out surveys or questionnaires on what they recall about particular behaviors, such as what foods they ate or what nutritional supplements they took in past years. Researchers don't change anything—they simply look at what is already going on. Such studies have most often tried to find connections between what people eat and the development of different diseases. A few have looked at the effect of taking nutritional supplements.

Observational studies are open to dispute and mixed interpretation by their very nature. For example, people with a well-balanced diet may also exercise more or take care of themselves better in other ways. The best studies aim to take these other possible contributing factors into account, but this can never be done completely.

Intervention Trials

An *intervention* trial tells us more than an observational study. In an intervention trial, researchers "intervene" in the participants' lives in some way to see what happens. This type of study is prospective—it follows people into the future.

In a *chemoprevention intervention* trial, for example, participants take a specific agent, such as a nutritional supplement, thought to help prevent a particular disease. They are then followed to see if they are less likely to get the disease than others not taking the agent. The best type of intervention trial uses a control group receiving a placebo (inactive pill), randomly assigns participants to the treatment and control groups, and uses the double-blind format in which neither researchers nor subjects know which treatment each participant receives.

However, intervention trials designed to show a reduction of cancer incidence are very difficult to do—they're expensive, require a long time period, and pose ethical questions (should you give people something that may make them develop more cancer?). Because of this, most evidence for cancer prevention has come from laboratory and animal models, and observational studies.

Intervention trials usually focus on high-risk groups of people rather than the population at large. One of the reasons for this is that a higher percentage will develop cancer, so it is possible to obtain meaningful results with a smaller total number of people. Also, it is easier to obtain funding for studies that aim to help people at great risk of a disease. It is for this reason that the first major chemoprevention intervention trials studied the effect of the antioxidants beta-carotene and vitamin E in smokers.

Studies of Nutrients

Observational studies of diet suggest that foods high in vitamin E, beta-carotene, and vitamin C provide strong preventive effects against a wide range of cancers. The much fewer studies of single nutrients in supplement form have not shown the same across-the-board benefit, but some of them have shown protective effects against specific cancers. It may be that a combination of nutrients—as found in natural dietary sources like fruits and vegetables—provides the greatest benefit.[2]

Foods high in vitamin E, beta-carotene, and vitamin C provide strong preventive effects against a wide range of cancers.

Of the nutrients in supplement form, vitamin E, selenium, and multivitamin formulations appear to be the most effective cancer preventives. Other vitamins and minerals believed to possess some degree of cancer-preventive effects include folic acid, vitamin D, calcium, and molybdenum. In this chapter, we'll look at the various nutrients in order of the relative weight of evidence for their benefits—from strongest to weakest evidence.

Vitamin E: Helpful Both As a Supplement and in Food

Vitamin E (tocopherol), a potent fat-soluble antioxidant, shows the strongest cancer-preventive evidence among the supplemental nutrients. Scientists think vitamin E may defend cell membranes and DNA against damage

caused by oxygen free radicals. Vitamin E also appears to bolster the immune system, which may play a significant role in cancer prevention.[3] Vitamin E and other antioxidants such as vitamin C, beta-carotene, and selenium appear to work as a team.[4]

> Of the nutrients in supplement form, vitamin E, selenium, and multivitamin formulations appear to be the most effective cancer preventives.

What Is the Scientific Evidence for Vitamin E?

Vitamin E in *supplement* form appears to significantly lower the risk of prostate cancer, as well as to protect against cancers of the colon, mouth, and throat. Consumption of vitamin-E rich *foods* is associated with a lower risk for cancers of the colon, stomach, mouth, throat, esophagus (food tube), liver, and breast (hereditary).[5]

What is the difference between vitamin E in supplement form and vitamin E in food form? Foods that contain vitamin E contain numerous other nutrients that may

A Note About Daily Value

On nutritional product labels you will see references to "DV." The new term *Daily Value* (DV) replaces the older term *Recommended Dietary Allowance* (RDA). These values are designed to meet or exceed most people's requirements for that nutrient, and represent, in most cases, a wide margin of safety. DVs are not minimal requirements—they contain an extra allowance for most groups of people.

provide benefits of their own. When you take vitamin E as a supplement, you get far more vitamin E than you are likely to get in food (10 to 50 times as much), but you don't get these other substances. The resulting effects are simply different. The following discussion distinguishes between foods high in vitamin E (dietary vitamin E) and vitamin E in supplement form.

All Cancers

Positive results for various cancers have been found for dietary vitamin E. In Finland, a study of 36,265 adults found that a diet low in vitamin E increased the overall cancer risk by 50%.[6] The risk varied for different cancer sites and was strongest for some digestive tract cancers and for the combined group of cancers unrelated to smoking. The association was strongest among nonsmoking men and among women with low blood levels of selenium. The results for women suggest that either low vitamin E or low selenium, or both, may play a role in increased cancer risk.

Positive results have also been found for vitamin E in supplement form. In a study of 11,178 elderly individuals (the group at highest cancer risk), those who reported taking vitamin E had a 59% reduction in cancer deaths. After adjustments for alcohol use, smoking history, aspirin use, and other medical conditions, the results still stood.[7] This study is among several demonstrating that a vitamin E supplement could also help prevent death from heart disease.

Prostate Cancer

Results from the Alpha-Tocopherol Beta-Carotene Cancer Prevention Study (ATBC), a major chemoprevention intervention trial, showed that vitamin E in supplement form exhibited a significant preventive effect against prostate cancer in men who smoked.[8] The trial had followed more than 29,000 male smokers in Finland who took supplements of either 50 mg of synthetic vitamin E (dl-alpha-tocopherol), 20 mg of beta-carotene, both, or a placebo (inactive pill) daily for 5 to 8 years.

Vitamin E supplements have been shown to lower the risk of cancers of the prostate, colon, mouth, and throat.

This study is exciting because it is an intervention trial in which participants took vitamin E supplements under controlled conditions.

Because the trial was primarily intended to look at the effect on lung cancer, all 29,133 participants were smokers. Vitamin E showed a marginal preventive effect against lung cancer, but the best news was for prostate cancer: Those taking 50 mg of dl-alpha-tocopherol (about 55 IU of synthetic vitamin E) daily for 5 to 8 years had a 32% lower incidence of prostate cancer and 41% fewer prostate cancer deaths.

Surprisingly, positive results came soon after the start of supplementation. Prostate cancer grows very slowly, and this suggests that vitamin E might block the progression of the disease to a more dangerous later stage.

This result is all the more impressive because vitamin E failed to prevent heart disease in this study. That further suggests that smoking may overwhelm vitamin E's preventive effect against heart disease more than it does against prostate cancer. It's possible that vitamin E supplementation may work even better in nonsmokers, but we don't know this for sure.

The dose of vitamin E used in this study is lower than that usually recommended. It is reasonable to think that a higher dose might be even more effective. Finally, a synthetic form of vitamin E was used in the study, which might not be the optimal form (see the sidebar, What Form of Supplemental Vitamin E Is Best?).

Colon Cancer

The ATBC study also found that vitamin E supplementation reduced the risk of colon cancer by 16%. Again, the ATBC study was a controlled intervention trial, the type of study that yields the most dependable results.

Another supplement study, though not an intervention trial, found vitamin E even more effective. Researchers at the Fred Hutchinson Cancer Research Center in Seattle determined that supplemental vitamin E (200 IU or more daily) cut colon cancer risk by 57% compared to those not taking vitamins.[9] Interestingly, a daily multivitamin supplement lowered the risk by almost as much—51%. The risk was also lowered in people taking supplements of vitamins A, C, folic acid, and calcium, but not as much.

The retrospective study looked at information on 444 patients with colon cancer and 427 control subjects over a 10-year period. Other risk factors, such as intake of vitamins from the diet, alcohol, fiber, and exercise, were taken into account. Still, the researchers pointed out the possibility that supplement users might be more likely to practice other preventive behaviors, and that more studies were needed to firm up the supplement connection. Any study not done under controlled conditions is susceptible to some uncertainties.

An analysis of the Iowa Women's Health Study Cohort found that foods high in vitamin E significantly reduced the risk of colon cancer in women under age 65. This effort was part of a larger study of breast cancer funded by the National Cancer Institute.[10] The study of 35,215 women ages 55 to 69 found that those with the highest dietary intake of vitamin E had the greatest protection. The protective effect was marginal for those over age 65. Results broke down like this: Women ages 55 to 59 showed the greatest benefit—an 84% lower risk; women ages 60 to 64 had a 63% lower risk; and women ages 65 to 69 had a 7% lower risk. Women under age 55 were not studied.

Cancers of the Mouth, Throat, Esophagus, and Stomach

Out of several vitamin and mineral supplements evaluated, vitamin E was the only one found to significantly reduce cancer risk in a population-based case-control study of oral and pharyngeal cancer in four areas of the United States.[11] Multivitamin supplements did not show a protective effect, while supplements of individual vitamins, including vitamins A, B, C, and E, were associated with a lower risk after controlling for the effects of tobacco, alcohol, and other risk factors for these cancers. After further adjustment for use of other supplements, vitamin E was the only supplement that showed a significantly reduced cancer risk. Smoking and drinking cause 75% of oral cancers, the researchers added, and avoiding these risk factors would lower the risk equally as well.

Studies of foods high in vitamin E have found similar positive results for cancers of the stomach, mouth, throat, and esophagus.[12]

Breast Cancer

An interesting 1995 study found that foods high in vitamin E were associated with a significantly decreased risk of breast cancer in premenopausal women with a family history of breast cancer.[13] The study involved 262 premenopausal and 371 postmenopausal women with breast cancer from western New York. The association was much weaker for women with no family history of breast cancer.

Though the results are promising, such a small, uncontrolled study has little statistical significance. In addition, the results were not published in one of the major journals regarded highly for rigorous scientific review (i.e., *New England Journal of Medicine, Lancet, Journal of the American Medical Association,* etc). But, if the results can be confirmed, they suggest that mechanisms of carcinogenesis may differ in women with and without a family history of breast cancer. Additionally, vitamin E may be a potential chemopreventive agent for women with a family history of breast cancer, particularly premenopausal women.

Dosage

The recommended daily value for vitamin E is 30 IU. The optimal dose of vitamin E for cancer prevention has not been determined, but a recent study analysis showed that 50 mg of synthetic vitamin E (about 55 IU) daily for 5 to 8 years reduced the incidence of prostate cancer by 32% and colon cancer by 16%. Heart disease studies show that at least 100 IU daily is required to reduce the risk of coronary heart disease, and that 400 and 800 IU daily had a strong preventive effect against nonfatal heart attack.[14] If you take vitamin E as a cancer preventive, it makes sense to take a dose that would also provide protection against heart disease.

You may see vitamin E doses listed in either international units (IU) or milligrams (mg). Converting between IU and mg can be confusing, because vitamin E comes in

What Form of Supplemental Vitamin E Is Best?

Determining the best form of vitamin E involves more than the natural versus synthetic question, but let's look at that issue first.

Taking 100 IU of synthetic vitamin E, for example, is supposed to be the same as taking 100 IU of natural vitamin E. However, a 1997 Japanese study reported that it took 400 IU of synthetic vitamin E to equal the blood levels obtained with just 150 IU of natural vitamin E.[15] The researchers concluded that natural vitamin E is almost three times more active in the body than the synthetic form, and that the natural form is therefore preferred for treating and preventing disease. Another study found similar results.[16]

How can you tell whether a product is synthetic or natural? Once you understand how to read the product label, it's easy. Vitamin E, like many other chemicals, comes in two mirror image forms—a right-handed (dextro or d) and a left-handed (levo or l) form. Synthetic vitamin E is made up of both forms, so has dl in its name (e.g., dl-alpha-tocopherol). Natural vitamin E comes in only the "d" form (e.g., "d"-alpha-tocopherol). That's all there is to it.

several forms. For that reason, most sources just say that 1 mg of vitamin E is equivalent to 1 IU. That's certainly simple, but only correct for the synthetic form. Here's a guide:

- Synthetic vitamin E (dl-alpha-tocopherol) = 1.1 IU per mg
- Natural vitamin E (in the form of d-alpha-tocopherol acetate) = 1.36 IU per mg

But there's another important issue. Most vitamin E supplements contain only alpha-tocopherol, while foods contain several different tocopherols, including alpha-tocopherol and gamma-tocopherol. The gamma form appears to be important also.

A 1997 study found that the alpha and gamma forms of vitamin E may work best when taken together and that both may be necessary for optimal antioxidant activity. Additionally, taking the alpha form alone appeared to decrease blood levels of the gamma form.[17]

These studies suggest that the optimal vitamin E supplement would be the natural "d" form containing a mixture of tocopherols (including alpha and gamma).

However, all the scientific evidence we have for the effectiveness of vitamin E supplements comes from studies using alpha-tocopherol, so at this point we have no direct confirmation that mixed tocopherols are better. Some manufacturers may create confusion by calling the dl mixture (synthetic vitamin E) "mixed tocopherols," so read product labels carefully.

- Natural vitamin E (in the form of d-alpha-tocopherol) = 1.49 IU per mg

Supplemental vitamin E may be absorbed better when taken with food. Diets that contain large amounts of polyunsaturated fatty acids increase the vitamin E requirement, and diets containing antioxidants decrease the requirement.[18]

Food sources, listed in order of higher to lower vitamin E content, include wheat germ oil, sunflower seeds and oil, almonds, hazelnuts, safflower oil, peanuts, cod-liver oil, peanut butter, corn oil, peanut oil, corn oil margarine, lobster, salmon, soybean oil, and pecans. Unlike with vitamin C and beta-carotene, it is more difficult to get large amounts of vitamin E from your diet (most people get 3 to 15 IU daily from the diet). Except for wheat germ oil (about 36 IU per tablespoon), other foods don't offer large amounts. The nuts and oils that do contain vitamin E are also high in fats. To get the amounts generally associated with significant antioxidant activity requires taking supplemental vitamin E.

Safety Issues

Vitamin E has an excellent safety record. Relatively large doses of vitamin E have been taken for extended periods without apparent harm.[19] Most adults tolerate doses of up to 1,000 IU daily without adverse effects.[20]

In the ATBC study, vitamin E, which has a blood-thinning effect, appeared to increase the number of deaths from hemorrhagic stroke (the type caused by a ruptured blood vessel that bleeds into the brain). Of 29,133 male cigarette smokers (ages 50 to 69), there were 66 deaths in the vitamin E group compared to 44 deaths in the group taking a placebo (inactive pill). On the other hand, vitamin E reduced the number of deaths from ischemic stroke, the more common type caused by an obstructed blood vessel to the brain, and this may outweigh the increased risk of hemorrhagic stroke.

Because vitamin E thins the blood, check with your physician if you take other blood thinners such as Coumadin (warfarin), aspirin, ibuprofen, or other similar medications. Taking them together may thin the blood too much and increase the risk for abnormal bleeding. People with bleeding disorders should also exercise care. Even people without these extra risk factors for bleeding should probably not take more than 800 IU daily except on physician advice. There are at least theoretical concerns that high-dose vitamin E should not be combined with other natural blood thinners, such as garlic and ginkgo.

Selenium Helpful As a Supplement

Selenium is a trace mineral that functions chiefly as a component of glutathione peroxidase, an antioxidant enzyme that works with vitamin E to help protect cell membranes from free radical damage.[21] Although most people get enough selenium from their diet, the soils in some areas of the country are low in this mineral. Evidence suggests that selenium supplements may protect against some forms of cancer.

What Is the Scientific Evidence for Selenium?

Selenium in supplement form has been associated with a lower risk of cancers of the prostate, colorectal, and lung, as well as a substantial reduction in cancer deaths. Dietary sources of selenium are associated with a lower risk for cancers of the esophagus and stomach.

After reviewing the cancer research on selenium, the Food and Nutrition Board's Committee on Diet and Health stated that "Low selenium intakes or decreased selenium concentrations in the blood are associated with increased risk of cancer in humans."[22] The National Research Council said, "A large accumulation of evidence indicates that supplementation of the diet or drinking water with selenium protects against tumors induced by a wide variety of chemical carcinogens."

Cancers of Prostate, Lung, Colon, and Rectum

Selenium shows promise in preventing prostate, lung, colon, and rectal cancers. In a large intervention trial, people who took supplemental selenium had a 37% decrease in prostate, colorectal, and lung cancers as well as a 50% reduction in cancer deaths.[23] That was the unexpected discovery of this 10-year trial on prevention of skin cancer, as reported in the *Journal of the American Medical Association*. As an intervention trial, this study carries more weight than uncontrolled observational trials.

The study was originally designed to see if selenium supplementation could lower the recurrence of basal cell and squamous cell cancers, the most common skin cancers, as two smaller studies had suggested. Selenium failed that test, but researchers were pleased with the unexpected good tidings. In the double-blind randomized trial of 1,312 patients with basal or squamous cell skin cancer, subjects took 200 mcg tablets of selenium daily as brewer's yeast or a placebo (inactive pill). No cases of selenium toxicity occurred. The news was so good that the blinded phase of the trial was stopped early to allow all participants to take selenium.

"Ours is the first study to show in a Western population that a nutritional supplement may reduce the risk of cancer," said head researcher Larry C. Clark, Ph.D., associate professor of epidemiology at the Arizona Cancer Center, University of Arizona College of Medicine, in Tucson. The evidence was convincing enough for researchers to recommend that people in the placebo group take selenium.

Selenium (in supplement form) has been associated with a 50% reduction in cancer deaths.

"We hope physicians will become more informed about selenium and appropriately counsel their high-risk patients," Clark said, but noted that more studies were needed before he would recommend a selenium supplement generally. Still, he said that these results "have given a more solid scientific basis for the patient who wants to take supplements because of their perceived high risk."

No reduction in cancers specific to women were found, but only a quarter of the study participants were women.

Breast Cancer

In studies involving women, the Nurses' Health Study analyzed toenail clippings (reflecting selenium intake) collected from 62,641 female nurses and found no link between selenium intake and cancer.[24] Similarly, a 3.3 year prospective Dutch study of 62,573 women found no associations between dietary selenium and breast cancer.[25]

What do these results mean? One possible interpretation is that selenium is not as important in women as in men. Another may be that the benefits of selenium depend on taking amounts greater than nutritional doses.

Dosage

The recommended daily value for selenium is 70 mcg in men and 50 to 55 mcg in women.[26] It is not difficult to obtain this level from the diet, and most multivitamin-mineral supplements contain selenium. A cancer-preventive dosage is undetermined, but the usual recommended supplemental dose is 50 to 200 mcg daily. In children this may be reduced to 1.6 mcg per pound of body weight.

Of the various sources of selenium, organic forms such as selenomethionine, selenium-rich yeast, and selenium-enriched garlic may be preferable to inorganic sodium selenite.[27]

Grains are an excellent food source of selenium. Food sources, in order of higher to lower selenium content (111 mcg to 39 mcg per 100 gram serving), are wheat germ, Brazil nuts, oats, whole-wheat bread, bran, barley, orange juice, turnips, garlic, brown rice. The amount in foods varies according to selenium content of the soil from which they come. Selenium is also found in water, meats, chicken, and seafood.[28]

Safety Issues

Long-term use of selenium at recommended doses in adults has been shown to be safe, and daily doses up to 350 mcg are believed to be harmless. At levels of 750 to 1,000 mcg daily, toxic effects may begin to emerge, such as GI distress, central nervous system changes, garlic-like breath odor, and loss of hair and fingernails.[29] In excessive doses, selenium may give rise to superoxide compounds, destructive forms of oxygen. However, this effect is fairly common with high doses of any antioxidant. The American Cancer Society currently does not recommend selenium supplementation.

There are no known drug interactions, but selenium absorption is reduced in the presence of heavy metals and high doses of vitamin C.

Beta-Carotene: Helpful in Food, but May Not Be As a Supplement

Much confusion has surrounded beta-carotene's effect on cancer. The important question is, does it prevent cancer or cause cancer? We'll look at the intriguing beta-carotene story in a minute.

Beta-carotene is a carotenoid that serves as a "provitamin" or precursor of vitamin A—it is not vitamin A itself. Our intake of beta-carotene comes from eating plant foods, and the body converts about one-sixth of dietary beta-carotene to vitamin A.[30] Beta-carotene is one of the pigments that gives vegetables like carrots and sweet potatoes their deep color.

Beta-carotene and other carotenoids function as antioxidants to neutralize free radicals and prevent the tissue damage they cause. Their antioxidant activity may counter the cell and DNA damage that lead to initiation of the cancer process. In addition, carotenoids promote enzymes that inhibit carcinogens and enhance white blood cell function.

What Is the Scientific Evidence for Beta-Carotene?

The beta-carotene story serves as a lesson in the perils of forming simplistic conclusions about how nutrients work. In the early 1980s, a review of the epidemiological (population) studies clearly showed that people who ate diets of fruits and vegetables high in beta-carotene had significant protection against cancer. The risk for several cancers was lowered, including lung cancer by as much as 70%, as well as cancers of the stomach, esophagus, lung, oral cavity and pharynx (throat), endometrium, pancreas, and colon.[31] Additionally, beta-carotene in supplement form appeared to substantially lower cancer risk in animal studies.[32]

Foods high in beta-carotene offer significant protection against cancer.

Ten years after the 1971 launch of the bold "war on cancer," which had made no real dent in the disease, the idea that a simple, affordable nutritional supplement might hold the key to power over cancer was highly compelling. It seemed that beta-carotene was a natural miracle nutrient, and that the Grail was close enough to touch. The National Cancer Institute eagerly funded chemoprevention intervention trials to evaluate beta-carotene supplements.

ATBC, CARET, Physicians' Health Study

Unfortunately, the anticancer bubble seemed to burst for beta-carotene in 1994, when the results of the first major intervention trial came in—the Alpha-Tocopherol, Beta-Carotene (ATBC) study. Apparently, beta-carotene supplementation did not prevent, but actually increased the risk of getting lung cancer by 18%.

The trial had followed more than 29,000 male smokers in Finland who took supplements of either 50 mg of synthetic vitamin E (dl-alpha-tocopherol), 20 mg of beta-carotene, both, or a placebo (inactive pill) daily for 5 to 8 years.

The men taking beta-carotene also had 23% more cases of prostate cancer and 25% more cases of stomach cancer. And the beta-carotene group had 13% more deaths from obstructive heart disease and all types of stroke combined. Because the results went bafflingly cross-grain to expectations, they were generally chalked up to a statistical fluke.

But in January 1996, researchers monitoring the Beta-Carotene and Retinol Efficacy Trial (CARET)—a different study—confirmed the prior bad news with more of their own: The beta-carotene supplemented group had 28% more cases of lung cancer and 46% more lung cancer deaths, as well as 17% more overall deaths.[33] This study involved smokers, former smokers, and workers exposed to asbestos. Alarmed, the National Cancer Institute pushed the brake pedal on the $42 million trial 21 months before it was finished. At about the same time, the 12-year Physicians' Health Study of 22,000 male physicians was finding that 50 mg of beta-carotene taken every other day had no effect at all—good or bad—on the risk of either cancer or heart disease.[34] In this study, only 11% of the participants were current smokers and 39% were ex-smokers.

In 1996, a further analysis of the ATBC trial indicated that the increased lung cancer effect appeared to be associated with heavier smoking and higher alcohol intake.[35]

A 1998 analysis of the ATBC trial found that the 23% increased risk for prostate cancer in men taking a beta-carotene supplement was not statistically significant and was limited to men who drank alcohol. Interestingly, men taking both beta-carotene and vitamin E had fewer cases of prostate cancer than those on placebo. This could suggest either an enhanced effect for the nutrients in combination, or that the beneficial effect of vitamin E overrides any harmful effect of beta-carotene.[36]

Despite the unsettled playing field, other beta-carotene trials continue. The Women's Antioxidant and Cardiovascular Study of 8,000 women at high risk for heart disease (but not cancer) is looking at beta-carotene, vitamin E, and vitamin C. Harvard researcher Jo Ann Manson, MD, said, "We haven't seen any evidence of harm from beta-carotene in these women, and there's good reason to believe beta-carotene may benefit them. But we're going to be monitoring the interim results very closely."[37]

The evidence suggests that a diet high in beta-carotene shows clear-cut benefits against cancer, but a beta-carotene supplement apparently does not. Is this a clanking contradiction? Not necessarily.

As stated earlier, there is a real difference between eating foods high in a specific nutrient and taking the nutrient alone in pill form. Foods that are high in beta-carotene also contain large amounts of other healthy substances, such as other carotenes. It is possible that beta-carotene may merely be a "marker" for a diet high in fruits and vegetables, and that other substances in these plant foods confer the cancer-preventive effect. Or, beta-carotene may be protective only in the presence of other substances found in fruits and vegetables—the "teamwork" concept.

A clue supporting the "marker" idea is that men with higher blood levels of beta-carotene (from dietary sources) at the start of the ATBC trial went on to have fewer lung cancers, regardless of which supplements they took during the study. This suggests that the benefit might

How to Get Your Beta-Carotene
Without Taking a Supplement

With the jury still out on the value of beta-carotene supplementation, you might wish to forego supplements and get this nutrient from your diet. There are enough foods high in beta-carotene to make it feasible to get recommended antioxidant amounts from diet alone. The various forms of each of the foods following are listed in order from higher to lower beta-carotene content followed by the range in IU. Example: 1/2 cup mashed sweet potato contains approximately 28,000 IU of beta-carotene.

Sweet potato: 1/2 cup mashed, 1 baked, or 1 cup canned; 16,000 to 28,000 IU

Carrot: 1 raw or 1/2 cup boiled slices; 19,150 to 20,250 IU

Spinach: 1/2 cup canned, frozen, or boiled; 7,300 to 9,400 IU (raw only 1,900 IU)

Mango: 1 medium; 8,100 IU

be coming from other dietary substances. Beta-carotene is only one member of the nutrient group called carotenoids, so why single it out as the hero?[38] Additionally, taking a beta-carotene supplement may promote deficiencies of other natural dietary carotenoids, which could reduce overall protective benefits.[39]

An ATBC trial researcher suggested that beta-carotene may act as a promoter of preexisting but latent tumors. Along that line, Susan Taylor Mayne and colleagues at Yale University School of Medicine suggested that, at high beta-carotene blood levels, cigarette smoke may interact directly with beta-carotene in the lungs to create pro-oxidative products as described earlier, and

Squash, butternut; $^1/_2$ cup boiled; 7,150 IU
Squash, winter; $^1/_2$ cup baked; 3,600 IU
Papaya: 1 medium; 6,100 IU
Cantaloupe: 1 cup; 5,200 IU
Turnip greens: $^1/_2$ cup boiled or $^1/_2$ cup raw; 2,150 to 4,000 IU
Mustard greens: $^1/_2$ cup frozen or $^1/_2$ cup boiled; 2,150 to 3,350 IU

You can get 50,000 IU (30 mg) of beta-carotene, for instance, from 1 cup of cooked sweet potatoes, 3 medium carrots, or 1 cup of cooked pumpkin. To get 25,000 IU (15 mg), eat half of a medium, cooked sweet potato, $^1/_2$ cup of cooked pumpkin, $1^1/_2$ medium carrots, $1^1/_2$ cups of cooked spinach, or 2 medium-sized mangoes. Or mix and match as you like.

these may then act as cancer promoters. Additionally, inflammation caused by asbestos in the lungs generates reactive oxygen and nitrogen compounds that might turn beta-carotene into a cancer promoter. Clearly, there is much we still do not know.

Early Cancer of the Oral Cavity and Esophagus
This prospective study (the type that goes forward in time) found that beta-carotene supplementation (90 mg daily) showed "fair efficacy" against early cancerous lesions of the oral cavity and esophagus called leukoplakia.[40] But this study was small, involving only 23 patients, and researchers stressed the need for additional research.

Table 4. Carotenoid Content* of Some Common Foods** (mcg)

	Beta-carotene	Lutein and Zeaxanthin	Lycopene
Broccoli, cooked	1,000	1,400	0
Brussels sprouts	370	1,000	0
Carrot, raw	5,700	190	0
Kale, cooked	3,050	14,250	0
Peach	90	12	0
Pink grapefruit	1,600	0	4,150
Spinach, raw	2,300	5,700	0
Tomato	640	125	3,800
Tomato juice	1,650	0	15,600

Source: Adapted from material compiled by the National Cancer Institute and the U.S. Department of Agriculture

Amounts of carotenoids are estimates based on averaged amounts (1 mcg = $^1/_{1,000}$ of a milligram)

**Each food listed is about one serving ($^1/_2$ to 1 cup)*

Cervical Cancer

Beta-carotene stalled the growth of cervical dysplasia cells—premalignant cells that may lead to cancer—in the laboratory.[41] However, results from phase III beta-carotene chemoprevention trials have been negative.[42]

A Beta-Carotene Consensus

In December, 1997, 23 scientists from 10 countries met at the International Agency for Research on Cancer (IARC) in Lyon, France, with the aim to evaluate whether supplements containing beta-carotene and other carotenoids worked to prevent cancer or other diseases. The verdict was not positive.[43]

"In none of these trials did the drug have a significant preventive effect," said Dr. Harris Vainio, chief of the

Chemoprevention Unit at IARC. "Moreover, when given to regularly smoking volunteers, it was shown to increase the risk of lung cancer and mortality from cardiovascular diseases." Until different results come in, the researchers recommended that carotenoid supplements not be promoted as having cancer-preventing effects, emphasizing instead a diet high in fresh fruits and vegetables, which has been shown to lower cancer risk.

In summary, there's currently not enough meaningful evidence that supplemental beta-carotene offers significant protection against cancer, and evidence shows it may be harmful in smokers and asbestos workers. Beta-carotene needs can easily be met through the diet, and it's probably best to get it this way until more is known.

Dosage

The recommended daily value for beta-carotene is not known and a possible cancer-preventive dosage is undetermined.

Food sources, in order of higher to lower beta-carotene content, include sweet potato, carrots, spinach, mango, butternut and winter squash, papaya, cantaloupe, turnip greens, and mustard greens. Other foods, in no particular order, are broccoli, pumpkin, yellow corn, kale, apricot, and tomato.[44]

One IU of beta-carotene equals 0.0006 mg. To convert, for example, 25,000 IU to mg, multiply by 0.0006 to get 15 mg. To convert 15 mg to IU, divide by 0.0006 to get 25,000 IU.

Safety Issues

High doses of beta-carotene do not lead to vitamin A toxicity and don't appear to be significantly toxic in the general population. The primary effect observed with high beta-carotene doses (or eating large amounts of colored fruits and vegetables) is a yellowing of the skin (carotene-mia) produced by the same mechanism that imparts a bright orange color to carrots, cantaloupes, and sweet potatoes. This harmless condition disappears rapidly after stopping intake.[45]

A beta-carotene supplement has the potential to cause liver problems in heavy drinkers of alcohol. As mentioned previously, chemoprevention trials suggest that beta-carotene in single-ingredient supplement form may have harmful effects in smokers, especially heavy smokers.

Carotenoids in Foods

Carotenoids like beta-carotene were traditionally viewed mainly as vitamin A precursors (agents converted by the body into vitamin A), but the 500 or so different carotenoids may have other important roles. None of the three supplement studies used a natural source of beta-carotene or a mixed carotenoid supplement. Fruits and vegetables provide a mix, as do some supplements from natural sources.[46] When you break down the carotenoid content of some common foods, intriguing possibilities come to mind, not the least of which is the realization of what you may be missing by relying on a beta-carotene pill alone (see table 4).

Vitamin C in Foods, Yes—
Supplements, Maybe

Vitamin C (ascorbic acid) is a potent water-soluble antioxidant. It complements the action of vitamin E, a fat-soluble antioxidant, and research suggests that a combination of antioxidants exerts an enhanced effect.[47]

Vitamin C also helps counter harmful effects of environmental contaminants and toxic chemicals, and inhibits formation of cancer-causing nitrosamine compounds.[48] (Nitrosamines are formed in the stomach after the ingestion of nitrates and nitrites, chemicals used in the curing of meats such as bacon and ham and as a preservative in sandwich meats.) All these actions have led researchers to examine whether vitamin C can be helpful in preventing cancer. As with beta-carotene, the evidence is better for foods containing vitamin C than for vitamin C supplements.

What Is the Scientific Evidence for Vitamin C?

Studies suggest that consuming *foods* high in vitamin C has a preventive effect against several cancers. These include cancers of the stomach, bladder, breast, cervix, colon and rectum, salivary gland, esophagus, larynx, pancreas, prostate, and lung, as well as leukemia and non-Hodgkin's lymphoma. Taking vitamin C *supplements* may have a preventive effect against bladder cancer but the evidence is contradictory. A combination of supplemental vitamin C and vitamin E appears to help protect against sunburn, which may indirectly prevent future skin cancer. Overall, there's no convincing evidence of a cancer-preventive effect for vitamin C in the form of supplements.

Most of the studies of vitamin C and cancer prevention involved dietary sources of vitamin C rather than vitamin C supplements. With dietary studies, as we've already noted with beta-carotene, you can't assume that vitamin C is the hero—it's possible that other plant substances such as flavonoids are equally or more important. Let's look at what the studies show.

All Cancers

Numerous dietary studies indicate that foods high in vitamin C protect against cancers of the stomach, bladder, breast, cervix, colon and rectum, salivary gland, esophagus, larynx, pancreas, prostate, and possibly lung, as well as leukemia and non-Hodgkin's lymphoma.[49] However, one study found that dietary vitamin C did not appear to play a role in prostate cancer.[50]

Of 46 dietary studies, 33 found significant protection, with high intake of foods rich in vitamin C providing about a twofold protective effect compared with low intake.[51]

Stomach Cancer

There is fairly strong evidence that foods high in vitamin C are associated with low rates of stomach cancer.[52] One way that vitamin C may work is by blocking the formation of cancer-causing nitrosamines in the stomach.

Bladder Cancer

One of the few studies of supplemental vitamin C demonstrated that 500 mg or more daily was associated with a lower incidence of bladder cancer.[53] However, another study found no benefit.[54]

Colon Cancer

In another study, 1,000 mg of supplemental vitamin C failed to prevent new colon cancers after the development of one colon cancer.[55]

Breast Cancer

In a large observational study, taking 500 mg or more of supplemental vitamin C daily for six years failed to significantly protect against breast cancer.[56] Another study found similar results.[57]

Skin Cancer

A small study did find that supplemental oral vitamin C—when combined with vitamin E—protected skin from sunburn. Each of ten people took a daily combination of 2,000 mg of vitamin C and 1,000 IU of natural vitamin E (d-alpha-tocopherol) or a placebo (inactive pill). The nutrient combination significantly reduced the sunburn reaction. This might protect against later skin cancer, although we have no direct evidence of that.[58]

Dosage

The recommended daily value for vitamin C in adults is 60 mg.[59] A possible cancer-preventive dosage is undetermined. It's easy to get the DV of 60 mg from your diet, and not that difficult to get even 500 mg this way.[60] (See the sidebar, What Is the Best Dose of Supplemental Vitamin C?)

Food sources, listed in order of higher to lower vitamin C content, include acerola, guava, strawberries, papaya, orange juice, lemon juice, and grapefruit juice. Other foods in no particular order: broccoli, brussels sprouts, cantaloupe, cauliflower, cranberry juice, honeydew melon, kiwi, mango, and tomato juice. The acerola fruit offers the biggest load of vitamin C by far, with the fresh juice containing about 1,300 mg of vitamin C per serving. A typical serving of the other foods in the ordered list provides about 40 to 242 mg of vitamin C each.

Safety Issues

Generally, vitamin C seems to be safe.[61] Some concerns have been raised about potential DNA injury when vitamin C is taken at a dose greater than 500 mg daily, but this idea is based on theoretical findings that have not yet been confirmed.

It has been stated that larger doses—over 1 g (1,000 mg) daily—can cause kidney stones, but recent studies cast doubt on this. In the large-scale Harvard Prospective Health Professional Follow-Up Study, those taking the most vitamin C (over 1,500 mg daily) had a lower risk of kidney stones than those taking the least amounts. However, individuals with a history of kidney stones and those

What Is the Best Dose of Supplemental Vitamin C?

Very large doses of vitamin C are often recommended by some proponents, but a recent study suggests that 200 mg may be the optimal daily dose.[62] At a 200-mg single dose, bioavailability (the body's ability to use it) was complete. It seems that about 200 mg a day saturates the body and most of any higher dose is simply washed out in the urine. The researchers concluded that the recommended daily value should be

with kidney failure who have a defect in vitamin C or oxalate metabolism should restrict daily vitamin C intake to approximately 100 mg.[63]

Large daily doses (4,000 mg or over) may result in loose stools or diarrhea. Diarrhea may occur starting at 500 mg, though it's usually only temporary. Cutting back on the dose may alleviate this side effect. At about 4,000 mg, persistent diarrhea may occur.

Vitamin C, an acid (ascorbic acid), can acidify the urine, which may diminish the effect of some medications. An acidic urine can also cause false results in diabetic urine tests. Frequent chewing of chewable-type vitamin C tablets may cause some wearing down of your teeth due to the acid content. One tip is to crush the chewable tablets, dissolve them in water, and drink that. Or switch to regular tablets that you swallow.

Folic Acid

Folic acid (folates), one of the B vitamins, may offer protective benefits against colorectal and cervical cancers.

Folic acid deficiency is the most common vitamin deficiency worldwide. During pregnancy, this deficiency is as-

increased to 200 mg (this much, they added, could be obtained from the diet), that safe doses of vitamin C are those less than 1,000 mg daily, and that vitamin C daily doses above 400 mg have no evident nutritional value. Although further research is indicated, this finding does appear to mean that there is no extra benefit in taking huge doses of vitamin C.

sociated with birth defects. Evidence suggests that folic acid supplementation also cuts the risk of heart disease by lowering homocysteine levels. It normally functions in concert with vitamin B_{12} in many body processes, such as DNA and protein synthesis, cell division, and development of the nervous system and fetus. Although there is not as much evidence as for antioxidants, folic acid is also a promising cancer-preventive nutrient.

What Is the Scientific Evidence for Folic Acid?

Adequate dietary folic acid may be protective against cervical cancer, as well as cancers of the colon, lung, and mouth,[64] but it is not known whether supplementary folic acid confers the same benefit. However, folic acid supplementation can help reverse cervical dysplasia in women taking oral contraceptives (a doctor's supervision is mandatory).

Cervical Cancer

A 1992 study found that folic acid deficiency may help cervical cancer get a start, but taking folic acid supplements does not alter the course of the disease once

Upcoming Information

A major French study is looking at whether antioxidants can prevent cancer and heart disease. This double-blind placebo-controlled trial of 12,735 adult men and women is important because it targets the general population rather than a high-risk population such as smokers. It was begun in 1994 and is expected to last 8 years. The doses used in this study are as follows: 30 mg vitamin E, 120 mg vitamin C, 6 mg beta-carotene, 100 mcg selenium, and 20 mg zinc.[65] Called the SU.VI.MAX study, it's a primary prevention trial using nutritional doses (one to three times the recommended daily values) rather than larger, pharmacologic doses.

it is established.[66] Studies have shown that folic acid supplementation can help reverse cervical dysplasia in women taking oral contraceptives, but not in the general population.[67]

Women with cervical dysplasia show a high incidence of general nutritional deficiencies, as high as 67% in one survey.[68] For this reason it makes sense to take a multivitamin–mineral supplement to see if it helps.

Colon Cancer

A Harvard study indicates that dietary folic acid may help prevent colorectal cancer.[69] Foods high in folic acid lowered the risk of colorectal adenoma (polyp precursors of cancer) by 34% in men and 37% in women compared to the lowest dietary folic acid intake. High alcohol intake combined with low folic acid intake further increased risk. The researchers said that these results support efforts to increase dietary folic acid in segments of the population having diets with low intakes of this nutrient.

In an accompanying editorial, Gladys Block, Ph.D., of the University of California–Berkeley, favored folic acid supplementation and fortification of foods with folic acid. She said that only 9% of Americans eat the recommended five or more daily servings of fruits and vegetables (good sources of folic acid).

Dosage

The recommended daily value for folic acid in adults is 400 mcg.[70] In addition to folic acid from the diet, women of child-bearing age should take an extra 400 mcg daily in supplement form to prevent neural tube birth defects such as spina bifida and anencephaly in their babies.

In order to help you get the folic acid you need, the U.S. government requires that breads and breakfast cereals be fortified with folic acid, so count that as part of your supplement intake. Be aware that amounts in these "fortified" foods vary, so read the labels. Some cereals contain all the extra folic acid needed. Most over-the-counter multivitamin products contain 400 mcg of folic acid.

Food sources, in order of higher to lower folic acid content, include brewer's yeast, black-eyed peas, soy flour, wheat germ, beef liver, soybeans, wheat bran, kidney beans, lima beans, asparagus, lentils, walnuts, fresh spinach, peanut butter, broccoli, whole wheat cereal, brussels sprouts, almonds, oatmeal, cabbage, avocado, green beans, corn, pecans, blackberries, and orange.[71]

Safety Issues

Toxicity is almost nonexistent because folic acid is water soluble and is rapidly eliminated from the body. Up to 15 mg has

Folic acid deficiency is the most common vitamin deficiency worldwide.

been given daily without toxic effects.[72] However, folic acid should not be taken in high doses without a doctor's evaluation, because it may mask the signs of vitamin B_{12} deficiency while irreversible nerve damage progresses.

Several drugs taken chronically may increase the need for folic acid. The anticonvulsant phenytoin (Dilantin) and related drugs may inhibit folic acid absorption.[73]

Vitamin D

Researchers have long suspected that vitamin D (calciferol) has inhibitory effects on cancerous cells in the laboratory, although the evidence for an anticancer effect in people is extremely weak. Still, some research suggests that the vitamin may play a preventive role in cancers of the breast, colon, prostate, and pancreas, and may also increase survival chances in women with advanced breast cancer.

What Is the Scientific Evidence for Vitamin D?

Vitamin D may have a protective effect against colon cancer partly due to its ability to increase calcium absorption by the body. Researchers think calcium may inhibit cell growth and reduce bile acid and fatty-acid irritation in the colon. Some evidence suggests that vitamin D can retard the growth of breast cancer cells and make cells become less cancerous.

Breast Cancer

Results of one small study suggested that body stores of vitamin D may be associated with survival chances in women with advanced breast cancer. "Thirteen women with normal or high levels of active vitamin D survived the 6-month test period but, sadly, in those with low levels, 5 out of 13 died within 6 months," said Professor Barbara Mawer of the Manchester Royal Infirmary in central

England.[74] However, it is not clear whether low vitamin D levels accelerated the breast cancer, or the breast cancer lowered levels of vitamin D.

A study comparing the health habits of 133 breast cancer patients with women who did not have the disease found that exposure to sunlight lowered the risk of breast cancer by 30 to 40% or more.[75] In reaction to sunlight exposure, the body manufactures vitamin D, which is thought to confer the protective effect.

Women who live in southern states are known to get breast cancer significantly less than those who live in the North. Some northern states don't get enough sun from November to February to make the required levels of vitamin D. "It's possible that all it takes is 10 or 15 minutes outside in bright sunlight to get a benefit," said Esther John, an epidemiologist at the Northern California Cancer Center. "And that's just casual exposure. The sunlight you get on your face and neck and arms and hands when you're regularly dressed." So while the exact dose of sunlight needed is not known, a brief outdoor stroll might do it. She said the amount needed to protect against breast cancer is probably not enough to cause skin damage. Sunscreens that block ultraviolet rays would also block the formation of vitamin D. However, we don't really know for sure if the benefits of sunlight are actually due to vitamin D. Other unrecognized factors may be involved.

Colon Cancer

In some studies, dietary sources of vitamin D intake were connected to a lower incidence of colon cancer.[76] Other studies, however, did not support these results.[77]

Cancer of the Pancreas

A synthetic form of vitamin D (EB1089) that has less of the calcium-raising effect of natural vitamin D is being tested on patients with cancer of the pancreas at St. George's

Hospital Medical School in London. Prior laboratory tests on cultured cells indicated that the compound promoted tumor cell death, but the researchers don't know yet whether it will work in humans. In animal studies, the compound reduced breast tumors up to 40% with no observed harmful effects on other cells.[78] This is very preliminary evidence.

Prostate Cancer

Men with two types of vitamin D receptor genes may have an increased risk for prostate cancer and taking extra vitamin D could theoretically be protective, according to a report in *Cancer Research*.[79] Researchers compared 108 cancer patients undergoing surgical removal of the prostate with 170 cancer-free men. They found that 22% of those with cancer had two copies of a particular vitamin D receptor gene, one from each parent, while only 8% of the cancer-free men had two. Vitamin D may help prevent cancer by plugging into these receptor genes. The inference seems to be that men with two receptor genes require more vitamin D to get a protective effect. "Different men have different risks of prostate cancer and this could be based, in part, on how their bodies utilize vitamin D," said lead researcher Dr. Jack A. Taylor.

Dosage

The recommended daily value for vitamin D in adults is 400 IU (600 IU for those over age 70).[80] Many older people fall short of this intake because they don't get enough vitamin D from sunshine or milk, and most foods don't contain much, so supplementation may be appropriate.

Food sources include milk, margarine, egg yolk, liver, tuna, salmon, mackerel, herring, and cod liver oil. Many dairy products and breakfast cereals are fortified with vitamin D. The body also manufactures vitamin D from the action of sunlight on the skin.

The two major forms of vitamin D are D_2 (ergocalciferol) and D_3 (cholecalciferol). Vitamin D_2 is the form used to fortify foods and the one used in most nutritional supplements, while vitamin D_3 is that obtained from sunlight and found naturally in foods.[81]

Safety Issues

Of all vitamins, vitamin D has the greatest risk for toxicity at higher doses. Continued doses of 50,000 IU or more daily may result in vitamin D poisoning, which causes excessive blood levels of calcium (hypercalcemia) and potentially serious side effects such as kidney stones. Common symptoms include appetite loss, nausea, weakness, constipation, and weight loss. Vitamin D toxicity is especially dangerous in patients taking the heart drug digitalis, because its toxic effects are enhanced by excessive calcium in the blood.[82]

Of all vitamins, vitamin D has the greatest risk for toxicity at higher doses.

Many dairy products and breakfast cereals are fortified with vitamin D, so read food labels.

Calcium and vitamin D work hand-in-hand. Without adequate amounts of vitamin D, the body does not absorb calcium properly. Too much vitamin D, however, can cause the body to lose calcium via the urine. It's a good idea to limit supplemental vitamin D to no more than 800 IU daily, except on the advice of a physician.

Molybdenum

Molybdenum is a trace mineral that functions as a component of enzymes such as those involved in the detoxification of alcohol.[83] Molybdenum may have a possible anticancer effect due to its neutralization effects on carcinogens, though evidence is minimal.

What Is the Scientific Evidence for Molybdenum?

Some research suggests that high-level supplementation of some micronutrients, including molybdenum, may be cancer-preventive.[84] Population studies in China indicate that molybdenum levels in soil correlate to the rates of esophageal cancer—the lower the soil levels, the higher the cancer rates.[85]Areas in the United States in which there is no molybdenum in the drinking water show a 30% increase in esophageal cancer.[86]

Dosage

The adult human requirement of molybdenum appears to be about 75 to 250 mcg daily, which is easily furnished by the average diet. Some multivitamin–mineral supplements contain molybdenum.[87]

Food sources, in order of higher to lower molybdenum content (155 mcg to 21 mcg per 100 g serving), include lentils, split peas, cauliflower, green peas, brewer's yeast, wheat germ, spinach, brown rice, garlic, oats, rye bread, corn, barley, whole wheat, potatoes, onions, peanuts, green beans. As with selenium, the amount in foods varies according to molybdenum content of the soil from which they come. The average diet supplies 50 to 500 mcg daily.[88]

Safety Issues

In ordinary amounts, molybdenum is relatively nontoxic. Excessive daily intake may cause gout-like symptoms in some people due to excessive uric acid production. A safe and adequate daily intake of 150 to 500 mcg has been estimated.[89]

Calcium

The mineral calcium is a major component of teeth and bones. It is essential for proper nervous system function, muscle contraction, and nerve conduction in the heart. Osteoporosis, a thinning of the bones, is associated with chronic calcium loss from bones. This is a common problem in postmenopausal women, because the loss of estrogen contributes to the rate of bone loss.[90]

Calcium's purported benefits in preventing colon cancer are questionable. Some researchers think calcium protects the colon lining from damaging compounds in the stool, especially bile acids and fatty-acids. It may also inhibit excessive division and turnover in cells lining the colon, a process thought to precede colon cancer.

What Is the Scientific Evidence for Calcium?

Despite the belief by some researchers that calcium might protect against colon cancer, numerous population studies have found only weak and insignificant effects in preventing this disease. Laboratory animal studies that show a cancer protective effect of calcium have simply not panned out in humans.[91]

A study by University of Arizona researchers found that people taking a calcium supplement had lower levels of bile acids than those taking a placebo (inactive pill). Bacteria in the colon turn bile acids into forms that are thought to promote colon cancer. People with colon polyps (which often become cancerous) were assigned to one of four groups: those taking 1,500 mg of calcium carbonate daily; those eating 2/3 cup of wheat bran cereal (a fiber source); those doing both in combination; a placebo group taking only 250 mg of calcium and eating a low-fiber cereal. After 9 months, measurements showed that people taking the calcium, wheat bran, or both had lower levels of bile acids than those in the placebo group. The

What Is the Best Form of Supplemental Calcium?

Choose a calcium supplement with care. Studies have found potentially harmful lead levels in some products. This is a special concern for children and pregnant women. Formulations of "natural" oyster shell, bone calcium, and dolomite (calcium–magnesium) tended to be the worst offenders.[92] Products with apparently safe lead levels were synthetic compounds such as calcium carbonates or USP-type tablets (such as refined calcium chelates).

Though the synthetic supplements appear to be lead-safe, they aren't all the same in terms of absorption by the body.[93]

combination of wheat bran and calcium was no better than either one alone. "It looks like the wheat bran helped more than the calcium, but the study wasn't big enough to tell," said the lead researcher.[94]

Dosage

The recommended daily value for calcium in adults is 1,000 mg, and for those over age 50 it is 1,200 mg.[95] Many people don't get this much in their diets, so a supplement can help (nonfat milk, for example, contains about 300 mg of calcium per 8-ounce serving). Supplemental calcium may be better absorbed when taken with food. A possible cancer-preventive dosage is undetermined.

Primary food sources are dairy products. Green leafy vegetables are also high in calcium. Food sources, from higher to lower content of calcium (1,090 mg to 32 mg per 100 g serving), include kelp, cheddar cheese, kale,

Calcium carbonate should be taken with meals, because absorption is increased by more acid in the stomach. The same is true for bone-meal (mostly calcium phosphate) and oyster shell (mostly calcium carbonate). Soluble products such as calcium citrate, calcium lactate, calcium gluconate, and calcium citrate malate may be preferable for older people, who might not produce as much stomach acid. However, you have to take quite a few of these pills to get the recommended daily amount of calcium. Ask your pharmacist if you need help choosing a calcium supplement.

turnip greens, almonds, brewer's yeast, parsley, brazil nuts, tofu, figs, buttermilk, yogurt, wheat bran, whole milk, olives, broccoli, cottage cheese, soybeans, pecans, wheat germ, peanuts, raisins, green snap beans, prunes, cabbage, oranges, celery, cashews, carrots, sweet potato, and brown rice.

Safety Issues
Daily doses of calcium above 2,000 mg can be harmful. Large amounts may increase the risk of kidney stones.[96] High calcium levels may inhibit the absorption of iron, zinc, and other minerals. Drugs known to lower calcium levels include aluminum-containing antacids, furosemide (a diuretic), cholestyramine, estrogen, and anticonvulsants such as phenytoin (Dilantin). Thiazide diuretics may increase calcium levels.

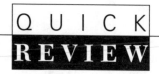

QUICK
REVIEW

- Vitamins C, E, beta-carotene, and the mineral selenium are antioxidants that neutralize free radicals, toxic compounds that can damage DNA and jumpstart cancer.

- Foods high in the antioxidant nutrients exert a strong cancer-preventive effect. Vitamin E and selenium carry the most evidence as cancer-preventive nutrients in supplement form. One study showed that a multivitamin supplement gave significant protection against colon cancer.

- There is a difference between getting your vitamins and other nutrients in food form versus taking them in supplement form. We have more evidence for the benefits of healthful foods than of supplements.

- Vitamin E may have the strongest protective credentials of all supplements. Taking a vitamin E supplement appears to significantly lower the risk of prostate cancer, as well as to protect against cancers of the colon, mouth, and throat. Foods high in vitamin E are associated with a lower risk for cancers of the colon, stomach, mouth, throat, esophagus, liver, and breast (hereditary). Suggested supplemental dosage: 100 to 400 IU.

- Selenium also has direct evidence backing it as a cancer preventive when taken as a supplement. Taking selenium supplements has been associated with a lower risk of cancers of the prostate, colorectal, and lung, as well as a 50% reduction in cancer deaths. Dietary sources of selenium are associated with a lower risk for cancers of the esophagus and stomach. Suggested supplemental dosage: 50 to 200 mcg.

- Foods high in beta-carotene appear to significantly lower the risk of cancers of the lung, stomach, esophagus, lung, oral cavity and pharynx, endometrium, pancreas, and colon. However, there is currently not enough meaningful evidence that supplemental beta-carotene offers significant protection against cancer, and it may be harmful in smokers and asbestos workers. Beta-carotene needs can easily be met through the diet, and it may be best to get it this way until more is known.

- Numerous studies indicate that vitamin C–rich foods may have a preventive effect on several cancers. These include cancers of the stomach, bladder, breast, cervix, colon and rectum, salivary gland, esophagus, larynx, pancreas, prostate, and lung, as well as leukemia and non-Hodgkin's lymphoma. But so far there is no convincing evidence that vitamin C in supplement form alone protects against cancer. Suggested supplemental dosage: at least 200 mg.

- Dietary folic acid may be protective against colorectal and cervical cancers, but it is not known whether supplementary folic acid confers the same benefit. However, folic acid supplementation can help reverse cervical dysplasia in women taking oral contraceptives.

- The evidence is minimal and less persuasive for the cancer-preventive benefits of vitamin D, molybdenum, and calcium.

- Keep in mind that, in studies of diets high in these nutrients, the observed cancer-preventive benefits could be due to other protective substances in the foods or to the combined effect of the nutrients working together. Studies showing little or no effect of supplemental beta-carotene and vitamin C lend weight to this view.

- A key point: Antioxidants in combination appear to work together to enhance overall benefit. With that in mind, it seems reasonable to take a combination of supplemental nutrients even though any single one may not be associated with a significant cancer-preventive effect. Such a regimen might include a comprehensive multivitamin–mineral formulation, vitamin E (100 to 400 IU), selenium (50 to 200 mcg), and vitamin C (at least 200 mg).

Phytochemicals That May Reduce Your Cancer Risk

Plant-based foods contain a hidden treasure of *phytochemicals,* a group of substances that may prove to be even more important than vitamins and minerals in preventing cancer and other diseases. Sometimes called *phytamins,* these bioactive compounds may not be essential to sustain life as are vitamins, but they may be essential to maintain a longer, healthier life.

The current frenzy of interest in phytochemicals can trace its origins back to obscure research on pellets of Purina rat chow.[1] In the 1960s, Lee Wattenberg, a researcher at the University of Minnesota, studied enzymes that protected animals from cancer. At first he thought that the animals' bodies probably maintained proper enzyme levels automatically. But when he switched them off their Purina diet, "The protection dropped to virtually zero in organs like the lung and the gastrointestinal tract," he said. The enzyme-stimulating ingredient turned out to be alfalfa meal. Later he discovered that phytochemicals called indoles found in vegetables like broccoli helped prevent breast and stomach cancers in animals.

"That was the prototype," Wattenberg said. "You could add constituents to an animal's diet and essentially protect against the development of cancer." Newer laboratory studies are deciphering how phytochemicals thwart carcinogenesis. "There is growing evidence that these natural products can take tumors and defuse them," said Devra Lee Davis, senior science adviser at the U. S. Public Health Service.[2] "They can turn off the proliferative process of cancer." "These compounds seem to interact with every step in the cancer process, mostly slowing, stopping, or reversing them," said John D. Potter, a cancer epidemiologist at the Fred Hutchinson Cancer Research Center in Seattle, Washington. These phytochemicals appear to increase the production or activity of enzymes that act as blocking agents or suppressing agents in the cancer process.[3]

Plant-based foods contain a hidden treasure of *phytochemicals* that may prove to be even more important than vitamins and minerals in preventing cancer and other diseases.

"Phytochemicals are the vitamins and minerals of the twenty-first century," said Mark Messina, Ph.D., a nutrition consultant and a former member of the National Cancer Institute staff, speaking at the annual research conference of the American Institute for Cancer Research. The industry, he said, may use phytochemical research to develop new prescription drugs—phytochemicals in concentrated forms for prevention of cancer in high-risk groups.

Phytochemicals and the exciting research on them is the focus of this section. The herbs and phytochemicals are presented in order of the relative weight of evidence for their benefits—from strongest to weakest evidence. This research field is still new, and more human studies are needed on all of these compounds. And, there are undoubtedly hundreds of other beneficial phytochemicals waiting to be discovered.

Tomatoes (Lycopene)

Lycopene, a carotenoid like beta-carotene, appears to exhibit approximately twice the antioxidant activity of beta-carotene and may exert stronger anticancer effects.[4] It's found in high levels in tomatoes and pink grapefruit.

What Is the Scientific Evidence for Lycopene?

Evidence is building that foods high in lycopene, such as tomatoes, may have a protective effect against cancer, including cancers of the esophagus, stomach, colon and rectum, prostate, and breast. Italian researchers studied people who ate tomatoes, which are much higher in lycopene than beta-carotene. Their results fit well with other studies, which found that one serving of raw tomatoes a week cut the risk of cancer of the esophagus by 40%. Elderly Americans consuming a diet high in tomatoes reduced their risk for cancers at all sites by 50%. Men and women who ate at least seven servings of tomatoes a week had lower risks of stomach and colorectal cancers compared to those who ate only two servings weekly.[5]

> **The industry may use phytochemical research to develop new prescription drugs.**

In a study of 48,000 male health professionals, Harvard Medical School researcher Edward Giovannucci and his team found significantly lower rates of prostate cancer among the men who ingested tomatoes, tomato sauce, or tomato-based foods such as pizza at least twice a week.[6] Men who never ate tomato sauce were up to 34% more likely to develop prostate cancer. Interestingly, tomato juice didn't help.

Elderly Americans consuming a diet high in tomatoes reduced their risk for cancers at all sites by 50%.

A tomato-rich diet may also help protect women against breast cancer. A study published in 1997 found that women with higher concentrations of lycopene and other carotenoids in their breast tissue were less likely to have breast cancer.[7]

Cooked tomatoes appear to be more bioavailable (more readily used by the body) than raw tomatoes, especially when the tomatoes are cooked in oil. "Probably what's happening is that the lycopene is in the cell walls, and it's hard to get at," said Giovannucci. "If you just eat a tomato, a lot of the lycopene passes through. But if you cook tomatoes in a little oil, then the cell walls break down with the heat, and the lycopene gets absorbed into the oil."

For the first time, researchers at Dana-Farber Cancer Institute in Boston have identified lycopene in prostate tissue samples from 25 men, according to a study published in the October 1996 issue of *Cancer Epidemiology, Biomarkers & Prevention*.[8] This does not prove that lycopene protects the prostate, but it does show that the prostate is a destination for the carotenoid.

A 1997 study of 1,300 European men showed that high dietary lycopene levels in the body cut the risk of heart attacks in half compared to low levels.[9]

Dosage

A cancer-preventive dosage of lycopene in humans is undetermined. Studies have shown apparent anticancer benefits for one to seven servings of tomatoes a week. Some commercial formulations may claim to offer the equivalent of one complete serving of fresh tomatoes.

Safety Issues

Dietary lycopene is assumed to be safe, since it is part of whole plant foods. Safety of concentrated lycopene in supplement form is not established, particularly in women who are pregnant or breastfeeding.

Soybeans (Isoflavone Phytoestrogens)

Isoflavone phytoestrogens are phytochemicals found in soybean and soy products like tofu (soybean curd) and non-dairy soy milk. One of the best known is named genistein. These substances are weak estrogen-like compounds that block the activity of the much stronger estrogen found in the human body naturally. Since breast cancer is partly dependent on estrogen, blocking the effect of this hormone inhibits the disease.[10] Genistein may also inhibit the formation of new blood vessels that feed tumors nutrients and oxygen, thus starving the tumors and stopping their growth.

What Is the Scientific Evidence for Soybeans?

Observational evidence suggests that people who regularly eat soy foods or products have a reduced risk of cancer of the breast, endometrium, prostate, colon, and perhaps other cancers.[11] However, it hasn't been proven that it is the soy foods in these diets that produce the protective benefits.

Certain substances present in soy do appear to exert anticancer effects, especially the isoflavone phytoestrogens such as genistein, which are found in high amounts in soybeans. Animal models show that genistein acts as an anti-estrogen, among other effects. In the lab, genistein suppresses the growth of a wide range of cancer cells.[12]

Evidence suggests that people who regularly eat soy foods have a reduced risk of cancer of the breast, endometrium, prostate, colon, and perhaps other cancers.

Researcher Stephen Barnes, Ph.D., a professor of pharmacology at the University of Alabama, is studying the effect of soy foods on breast and prostate cancer.[13] He's found that genistein appears to be far more potent in stopping cancer growth in normal cells than in cells which have already turned cancerous. In lab trials at the University of Alabama, genistein appeared to halt the proliferation of prostate cancer cells. The results were so promising that men were enrolled in clinical trials of soy protein powder as a possible prostate cancer preventive. The participants were 80 men with elevated levels of prostate specific antigen (PSA). Higher PSA levels are linked to higher prostate cancer rates.

A 1994 review study examined laboratory, animal, and population data.[14] Of the 26 animal studies involving diets containing soy or soybean isoflavones, 17 (65%) reported cancer-protective effects. Although population studies have been inconsistent, soy milk and tofu appeared to have protective effects against both hormone- and non-hormone-related cancers.

A 1997 Hawaiian study published in the *American Journal of Epidemiology* found that women who regularly ate the most soy foods such as tofu, soy milk, and roasted soy nuts cut their risk of endometrial cancer by more than half compared to women who ate none. In Asia, where most women eat soy regularly, rates of endometrial cancer are lower than in the United States.[15] Of course, there are many other differences in lifestyle between the United States and Asia, and it is not clear which factors are most important.

In an Australian study, women who ate foods high in phytoestrogens had a significantly lower risk of breast cancer, according to a report in *Lancet*.[16] Several earlier studies had suggested that these compounds might lower the risk of breast cancer. Ingram and colleagues at Queen Elizabeth II Medical Centre in Perth studied 144 women ages 30 to 84 who were newly diagnosed with breast cancer along with an equal number of women without cancer.

Green tea polyphenols have shown more potent antioxidant activity than either vitamin E or vitamin C.

By analyzing the women's urine for concentrations of two types of phytoestrogens, lignans and isoflavonoids, researchers could determine the amounts of phytoestrogen-containing foods they ate. The women whose diets were lowest in phytoestrogens—particularly the isoflavone equol and the lignan enterolactone—were significantly more likely to have breast cancer compared to those with the highest intake.

Of the numerous studies showing that diet plays a cancer-preventive role, not one of them "has shown a degree of risk reduction similar to that found for some phytoestrogens in this study," Ingram's team said. This means that certain phytoestrogens may be more powerful at reducing cancer risk than other aspects of the diet.

Dosage

Right now, no cancer-preventive dosage in humans for soy or extracted soy isoflavones has been determined. However, typical recommendations for soy foods suggest that one to two servings of soy daily produce a beneficial effect, while concentrated soy isoflavones can be taken at a dose of 40 to 60 mg daily.

Safety Issues

Dietary soy is believed to be safe, although high amounts can interfere with mineral absorption. Safety of concentrated isoflavones in supplement form is not established, particularly in pregnancy or breast-feeding. Individuals allergic to soy products should not use them.

Green Tea (Polyphenol Flavonoids)

Green tea polyphenols have shown more potent antioxidant activity than either vitamin E or vitamin C. Both green tea and black tea come from the tea plant called *Camellia sinensis*, which has been cultivated in China for centuries. More black tea is produced than green tea. The key difference between the two is in preparation. Black tea is prepared by drying and fermenting the leaves. This tea is most widely consumed in Europe, India, and North America. Green tea is not fermented and is made by steaming or pan-frying tea leaves and then drying them. It is consumed mostly in China and Japan, where it has been used medicinally as a stimulant and digestive remedy for about five thousand years.[17]

What Is the Scientific Evidence for Green Tea?

Laboratory and animal studies have shown that tea consumption protects against cancers of the stomach, lung, esophagus, duodenum, pancreas, liver, breast, colon, and rectum.[18] However, results from human studies have not been so clear-cut—some have shown a protective effect and others have not. The overall weight of evidence does lean toward the positive side.[19]

Traditionally, Americans drink black tea and Asians drink green tea. Most of the research news has been about the possible cancer-preventive effects of green tea.

In animal studies, green tea polyphenols stimulate the activity of antioxidant and detoxifying enzymes in the lungs, liver, and small intestine.[20] Polyphenols may also block the formation of nitrosamines and other cancer-causing compounds as well as trap or detoxify carcinogens. Nitrosamines form when nitrites bind to amino acids. Nitrites are used in the curing of meats such as bacon and ham and as a preservative in sandwich meats.[21]

In one of two groundwork studies in Ohio, researchers at the Medical College of Ohio found that the green tea flavonoid EGCG binds and deactivates an enzyme called urokinase, which has been shown to play an important role in the growth and spread of malignant tumors. Mice showed reductions in tumor size and even complete remissions. At Case Western University, researcher Hasan Mukhtar, Ph.D., discovered that the combination of green tea flavonoids epicatechin-3 gallate (ECG) and EGCG "selectively destroys cancerous cells while sparing healthy ones."[22]

A 1994 study of skin cancer in mice found that both black and green teas, even decaffeinated versions, inhibited skin cancer in mice exposed to ultraviolet light and other carcinogens.[23] After 31 weeks, mice given the teas brewed at the same concentration humans drink had 72 to 93% fewer skin tumors than mice given only water. In an earlier Swedish study, drinkers of black tea had a significantly lower rate of stomach cancer.

Human studies, as mentioned, have shown varied results. One study followed 8,552 Japanese adults for nine years. Females who drank more than 10 cups a day had a delay in onset of cancer and also a 43% lower cancer incidence. Males had a 32% lower cancer incidence, but researchers said this was not statistically significant.[24]

Another study reviewed the population studies on the effect of tea drinking on stomach, colon, and lung cancer as well as overall cancers.[25] Researchers found no protective effect of tea on stomach cancer and on the total risk of cancer. Green tea showed some evidence of having a protective effect against colon cancer. There was also modest evidence that regular use of black tea might lower the risk of colon and rectal cancers. Surprisingly, some studies suggested an increased risk of lung cancer with increased tea consumption. The researchers pointed out that flaws can creep into population studies such as these and influence results. The conclusion was that any positive benefit suggested by the limited studies was likely restricted to high intakes in high-risk populations.

A study in Shanghai, China, found that those who drank green tea had significant reductions in the risk of developing cancer of the rectum and pancreas. There was no significant decrease in colon cancer.[26] A total of 3,818 residents ages 30 to 74 were included in the population study. For men, those who drank the most tea had a 28% lower incidence of rectal cancer and a 37% lower incidence of pancreatic cancer compared with those who did not drink tea regularly. For women, the respective lower cancer incidences were even greater—43% and 47%.

Another study in Shanghai, China found similar results for stomach cancer. Green tea drinkers were 29% less likely to get stomach cancer than nondrinkers, with those drinking the most tea having the least risk.[27] Interestingly, the risk of stomach cancer did not depend on the person's age when green-tea drinking started. Researchers suggested that green tea may disrupt the cancer process at both the intermediate and late stages.

Texas Medical Center cancer researchers are currently seeking more definitive information about the effect of green tea on cancer.[28] "The epidemiologic studies are interesting," said Waun Ki Hong, M.D., of the University of Texas M.D. Anderson Cancer Center in Houston. "In Japan, people who drink green tea have a delayed occurrence of cancer compared to those who don't drink it."

The phase I trial to determine green tea's safety, side effects, and toxicity will include 30 patients with advanced cancer of the lung, breast, prostate, ovaries, or head and neck. Patients will take capsules of green tea extract equivalent to 6 or 7 cups. Hong thinks the supplement will prove effective at preventing cancer but not at treating it.

Dosage

A cancer-preventive dosage of green tea in humans is not known. For medicinal use, 5 to 10 ml of the dried herb is steeped in a cup of boiling water for about 15 minutes. The usual amount taken is 1 to 3 cups daily, without the addition of milk or sugar. More recently, green tea capsules have been developed for the market, but the clinical benefits of these are unknown.[29]

Safety Issues

No adverse effects have been reported for the medicinal use of green tea. However, a cup of tea, black or green, contains 10 to 80 mg of caffeine, depending on the methods used in its production, storage, and preparation. Excess caffeine can cause nervousness, insomnia, and irregularities in heart rate. Extensive safety studies have not been performed and safety in pregnancy and breast-feeding has not been established. Pregnant women, breast-feeding mothers, and patients with cardiac problems are usually advised to limit their intake to two cups daily.[30]

Garlic and Onion (Organosulfides)

Animal and test-tube experiments show that compounds present in garlic and onion inhibit the growth of cancer-ous tumors. Studies suggest, but do not prove, that dietary garlic and onion may protect against cancers of the colon and stomach in humans, and possibly other cancers.

Garlic and onion (as well as chives and scallions) be-long to the allium family of plants. Garlic does not grow in the wild, but has been cultivated and widely ingested as a food for centuries. The unique odor associated with gar-lic—imparted by its sulfur compounds—may occur to an extent even in "odorless" formulations, perhaps due to conversion of alliin to allicin in the digestive tract. The odor may serve to ward off insects.[31]

What Is the Scientific Evidence for Garlic and Onion?

The mechanism for the anticancer effects is not known, but researchers speculate that one way garlic may work is by killing bacteria in the stomach that help promote the formation of cancer-causing substances in the gastrointesti-nal tract.[32] Selenium from the soil also exerts anticancer ef-fects, and one reason for the cancer-preventive effects of garlic and onion may be the high levels of selenium they contain.[33] (See the discussion of selenium in chapter 5.)

Garlic

In animal studies, garlic extract and allicin have exhibited potent antitumor effects. Population studies in China, Italy, and the United States have shown that diets high in garlic may confer a cancer-protective effect.[34]

The Iowa Women's Study, one of the best population studies, followed 41,837 women for several years. At the start, women filled out questionnaires about their lifestyle habits. After 4 years, follow-up questionnaires showed that the women who ate significant amounts of garlic lowered their risk of colon cancer by 32%.[35]

A study in mice offers promise that garlic may help protect against lung cancer. At Queen's University in Kingston, Ontario, Poh-Gek Forkert, a cellular toxicologist administered a garlic derivative (diallyl sulfone) to mice and exposed them to a chemical carcinogen that affects lung tissue. The chemical had no effect on the lungs of garlic-treated mice, but severely damaged the lungs of mice not given garlic.[36] With funding from the National Cancer Institute, Forkert plans further research on the possible protective effects of garlic on samples of mice and human lung tissue. "Since we've been doing this work," she said, "everybody in the lab has been eating a lot of garlic just in case."

Onion

An onion extract (diallyl disulfide) killed tumor cells in the laboratory and stalled growth of tumor cells implanted in rats, inhibiting colon and kidney cancers.[37]

Eating at least half an onion daily lowered the risk of stomach cancer by half, according to the Netherlands Cohort Study on diet and cancer.[38] Researchers followed 120,852 men and women ages 55 to 69 for more than 3 years. Interestingly, the use of garlic supplements was not associated with reduced stomach cancer risk.

Dosage

It is unclear how much garlic or onion is needed for a cancer-preventive effect in humans. A typical medicinal daily dose of garlic might be 2 to 5 g of fresh garlic clove or its equivalent.[39] For onion, typical daily doses would be equivalent to 2 to 5 ounces of fresh onion (about ¼ cup to 1 cup of chopped onions).[40] It is not clear whether dried, powdered garlic supplements sold for the purpose of lowering cholesterol would have the same effect as whole garlic.[41]

Safety Issues

Other than bad breath, in some cases garlic can cause gastrointestinal disturbances such as heartburn or flatulence (gas). There have also been occasional reports of allergic reactions. Garlic appears to have a blood thinning effect, so do not combine it with blood thinning drugs such as warfarin (Coumadin) or heparin except under the supervision of a physician. No significant toxicity has been reported for onion.[42] There are least theoretical concerns that garlic should not be combined with other natural blood thinners, such as high-dose vitamin E and ginkgo.

Flaxseed Oil (Lignans)

Flaxseed is a high-fiber grain that has been cultivated since ancient Egyptian times. It is an abundant source of lignans, a precursor of certain phytoestrogens, which have anticancer effects. Flaxseed oil is also a rich source of omega-3 fatty acids and contains both the essential fatty acids, alpha-linolenic acid (an omega-3 fatty acid) and linoleic acid (an omega-6 fatty acid).[43]

What Is the Scientific Evidence for Flaxseed Oil?

Studies in both animals and humans have shown that lignans may protect against cancer, especially breast cancer. One way lignans may exert their proposed anticancer effects is by being converted into phytoestrogens such as enterolactone and enterodiol in the body. Phytoestrogens are weak estrogen-like compounds that block the activity of the stronger estrogen found naturally in the body. Since breast cancer is partly dependent on estrogen, drugs that block the effect of the hormone can inhibit the disease.[44] Lignans may be able to do so as well, although this has not been proven.

Feeding rats flaxseed flour after giving them a known carcinogen resulted in a 67% reduction in the size of breast tumors that formed.[45]

In an Australian study, women who ate foods high in the lignan enterolactone had a significantly lower risk of breast cancer, according to a report in *Lancet*.[46] The study included 144 women ages 30 to 84 who were newly diagnosed with breast cancer along with an equal number of women without cancer.

The alpha-linolenic acid in flaxseed oil showed anti-cancer activity, especially against breast cancer, according to a study of 121 women with the disease. Low levels of alpha-linolenic acid in breast fatty tissues was associated with an increase in cancer invasiveness and its spread (metastasis) to other areas of the body.[47]

Dosage

The proper cancer-preventive dosage of flaxseed in humans is as yet undetermined. The typical supplemental dose recommended by some nutritionists is 1 to 2 tablespoons of flaxseed oil daily. Flaxseed oil is easily damaged by heat and light, so don't cook with it. The most palatable way to take it is by adding it to foods, such as using it as a salad dressing.[48]

Safety Issues

Flaxseed oil is thought to be safe in nutritional amounts (for example, 1 to 2 tablespoons daily).

Licorice

The anti-inflammatory effects of licorice *(Glycyrrhiza glabra)* may play a role in its purported cancer-preventive effects. Licorice is a perennial herb or subshrub, and licorice root has a long history of medicinal use including the treatment of malaria, peptic ulcers, asthma, pharyngitis, insomnia, abdominal pain, and microbial infections. Licorice is widely used as a flavoring agent. Of the over 200 phytochemicals so far identified in licorice, about 29 may have biological activity against cancer. Flavonoids, coumarins, tri-terpenes, and phenolic acid appear to be the most promising.[49]

Stronger Neominophagen C, a licorice-derived formulation used in the study discussed following, appears to protect the liver cell membrane from damage. This action may also explain its ability to lower elevated levels of the liver enzyme ALT in patients with chronic hepatitis. The National Cancer Institute is currently evaluating the liver protective effects of licorice as well as its possible role in slowing cell mutations.[50]

However, there is no direct evidence that oral licorice can affect cancer. Furthermore, long-term use of licorice can cause numerous health problems (see Safety Issues).

What Is the Scientific Evidence for Licorice?

Although study results must be regarded as preliminary, a licorice-derived intravenous solution, Stronger Neominophagen C (SNMC), showed a significant preventive effect on liver cancer in patients with chronic hepatitis C, according to a Japanese study.[51] Infection with the hepatitis C virus may play a role in the majority of cases of liver cancer (hepatocellular carcinoma). SNMC is composed of glycyrrhizin, cysteine, and glycine. Glycyrrhizin is an aqueous extract of licorice root.

This retrospective study examined the hospital records of 453 patients diagnosed with chronic hepatitis C. Researchers determined that 84 patients had been treated with SNMC given at a dose of 100 ml daily for 8 weeks, then 2 to 7 times weekly for 2 to 16 years. It turned out that the patients who had not been given SNMC were two-and-a-half times more likely to get liver cancer. Additionally, the long-term administration of SNMC tended to normalize levels of the liver enzyme ALT, which the authors concluded may indicate a protective effect against liver cancer.

Dosage

A cancer-preventive dosage in humans is undetermined, but the following are typical licorice dosages (given 3 times daily):[52]

> Powdered root: 1 to 2 g
> Fluid extract (1:1): 2 to 4 ml
> Solid (dry powdered) extract (5% glycyrrhetinic acid): 250 to 500 mg

Warning: Licorice can cause severe side effects when taken long term. Additionally, do not attempt to inject licorice products designed for oral use.

Safety Issues

The chemical structure of licorice is similar to the corticosteroids (the body's adrenal gland hormones), and it has similar effects. Consuming over 3 g of licorice root daily for more than 6 weeks may cause electrolyte imbalances, fluid retention, irregular heart rhythms, and elevated blood pressure. Licorice should be avoided by individuals taking digitalis heart medications and those who have high blood pressure or kidney failure, except under medical supervision.[53] Safety in pregnancy and breastfeeding has not been established.

Ginseng

Panax ginseng, also known as Korean or Chinese ginseng, is the most popular of several types of ginseng. Wild ginseng is rare, but it is cultivated in several countries. Ginseng has a long history as a folk medicine, and is used for almost every conceivable condition. Based on its traditional mystique, ginseng has been suggested as a treatment for cancer as well. For more information on ginseng, see *The Natural Pharmacist: Your Complete Guide to Herbs*.

What Is the Scientific Evidence for Ginseng?

According to an observational study of 905 individuals in Korea, regular consumption of ginseng appeared to significantly lower the risk of cancers.[54]

A greater anticancer effect was seen with ginseng extract and powder than with fresh sliced ginseng, ginseng juice, or ginseng tea. There was a dose–response relationship, meaning the greater the dose, the greater the anticancer effect.

However, this preliminary research needs to be followed up by more reliable studies before we can consider ginseng to have proven anti-cancer benefits.

Dosage

The typical dose of ginseng is 1 to 2 g of root daily or 100 to 300 mg of extract (standardized to contain 7% ginsenosides) 3 times daily taken for 3 to 4 weeks.[55]

Safety Issues

The various forms of ginseng appear to be nontoxic, both in the short and long term, according to the results of studies in mice, rats, chickens, and dwarf pigs. Ginseng also does not seem to be carcinogenic.[56]

Side effects are rare. Occasionally women report menstrual abnormalities and/or breast tenderness when they take ginseng, and overstimulation and insomnia have also been reported. Unconfirmed reports suggest that highly excessive doses of ginseng can raise blood pressure, increase heart rate, and possibly cause other significant effects. Whether some of these cases were actually caused by caffeine mixed in with ginseng remains unclear. Ginseng allergy can also occur, as can allergy to any other substance.

In 1979, an article was published in the *Journal of the American Medical Association* claiming that people can become addicted to ginseng and develop blood-pressure elevation, nervousness, sleeplessness, diarrhea, and hypersexuality. This report has since been thoroughly discredited and should no longer be taken seriously.[57]

However, there is some evidence that ginseng can interfere with drug metabolism, specifically drugs broken down by the cytochrome P450 enzyme CYP3A4. Ask your physician or pharmacist whether you are taking any medications of this type. There have also been specific reports of ginseng interacting with MAO inhibitor drugs and digitalis, although again it is not clear whether it was the ginseng or a contaminant that caused the problem.

Safety in young children, pregnant or breastfeeding women, or those with severe liver or kidney disease has not been established. Interestingly, Chinese tradition suggests that ginseng should not be used during pregnancy or lactation.

Lactobacilli

Lactobacilli is a "probiotic" composed of "friendly bacteria" normally present in the GI tract. Administration of prescription antibiotics often allows microbial overgrowth causing diarrhea, yeast infection, or urinary tract infection. Ingesting certain brands of yogurt containing the

L. acidophilus lactobacilli or a commercial formulation of *L. acidophilus* may help prevent or correct these conditions.[58]

Limited evidence suggests that lactobacilli may help prevent bladder cancer, but more studies are needed to confirm these results and also to see if lactobacilli formulations might have a preventive effect against other cancers.

What Is the Scientific Evidence for Lactobacilli?

Various laboratory studies have suggested that *L. bulgaricus*, the chief lactobacilli used in yogurt, can neutralize bacterial enzymes associated with the formation of cancer-causing compounds in the gut.[59] In human patients, formulations were effective in preventing recurrence of superficial bladder cancers.[60]

Dosage

A typical dose of lactobacilli is 2 to 3 capsules or tablets (or 2 to 3 billion CFU) 3 times daily before meals.[61] Yogurt is also a source of lactobacilli.

Safety Issues

Probiotics do not appear to be associated with significant risks or side effects.

Melatonin

Melatonin, a hormone produced by the pineal gland, is believed to play a key role in regulating the body's circadian rhythms and the sleeping/waking pattern. Researchers discovered that people produce higher levels of melatonin at night.[62] There is no convincing evidence that melatonin acts as a cancer preventive in humans.

What Is the Scientific Evidence for Melatonin?

The way melatonin might affect the proliferation of cancer cells is mostly unknown.[63] In test tubes, melatonin inhibits various cancers, especially those related to hormones such as breast cancer and prostate cancer.[64] Melatonin may be of value when added to standard combined chemotherapy of cancer, because it may augment the anticancer action and decrease the side effects of many chemotherapeutic drugs.[65] However, much more research is necessary.

Dosage

Typical doses of melatonin when used for sleep are 0.5 to 5 mg daily.

Safety Issues

The safety of long-term use of melatonin is unknown. Keep in mind that this is a hormone, not a dietary supplement. It's probably best not to take melatonin except on the advice of a physician.

Turmeric and Curcumin

Turmeric (*Curcuma longa*) is a perennial herb in the ginger family that is cultivated in China, India, Indonesia, and other countries. Turmeric is the chief ingredient of curry powder and is also used in prepared mustard. The herb is used in Chinese and Indian medicine as an anti-inflammatory agent and in the treatment of a wide range of conditions such as flatulence (gas), jaundice, menstrual irregularities, and toothache. There is some laboratory evidence that turmeric and its chief constituent curcumin may be of value in preventing cancer. However, human studies are needed to see if the laboratory promise of turmeric and curcumin translates to people.

What Is the Scientific Evidence for Turmeric and Curcumin?

Curcumin inhibits tumor development during both initiation and promotion periods in several experimental animal models.[66]

In mice, dietary curcumin appears to inhibit stomach, duodenal, and colon cancer, but has little or no effect on lung or breast cancer. Poor circulating bioavailability (availability to the body) of curcumin may account for its lack of activity against lung and breast cancer.[67]

Dosage

A typical dose of curcumin is 400 to 600 mg 3 times daily.

Safety Issues

Extensive safety studies of concentrated curcumin have not been performed. Safety is not established in women who are pregnant or breast-feeding.

Berberine (Goldenseal)

Berberine is the main berberis alkaloid found in the plants goldenseal, barberry, Oregon grape, and goldthread. These plants have been used for infections of the skin and digestive tract, gallbladder inflammation, and liver cirrhosis.[68] Berberine appears to kill tumor cells and also to enhance immune system function by stimulating white blood cells.[69] However, without adequate human studies, there is no way of knowing whether berberine has a significant cancer-preventive effect in people (for more information about berberine, see Goldenseal in the *The Natural Pharmacist: Your Complete Guide to Herbs*).

What Is the Scientific Evidence for Berberine?

In laboratory studies, berberine has demonstrated anti-cancer activity against malignant brain tumors in both rats and humans.[70] For brain tumor cells, berberine at a dose of 150 mcg/ml showed a cell kill rate of 91%. In comparison, the cell kill rate was 43% for BCNU, the standard chemotherapeutic agent for brain tumors. In rats with brain tumors, berberine at 10 mg/kg showed a cell kill rate of 81%. Combining the two agents was even more effective.

Dosage

A possible cancer-preventive dosage for berberine in humans is unknown. For goldenseal, typical doses are 0.5 to 1 g of the dried root or 2 to 4 ml of tincture (1:10, 60% ethanol) 3 times daily.[71]

Safety Issues

At normal doses, goldenseal does not seem to cause any obvious side effects. Excessive doses may cause nausea, vomiting, diarrhea, CNS stimulation, and respiratory failure. Goldenseal is contraindicated during pregnancy, and safety is not established in breast-feeding.[72]

Bromelain

Bromelain, derived from the pineapple plant *(Ananas comusus),* is composed of sulfur-containing enzymes that digest protein. It has been used for inflammation, sports injuries, painful menstruation, and respiratory tract infections.[73] Highly preliminary evidence from animal studies suggests that bromelain may also help prevent cancer.

What Is the Scientific Evidence for Bromelain?

In mice, bromelain delays the development of UV light-induced skin cancer and inhibits metastasis of the Lewis lung cancer. The lack of convincing studies in humans makes bromelain only a theoretical cancer preventive.[74]

Dosage

A typical dosage of bromelain is 250 to 500 mg 3 times daily between meals.[75]

Safety Issues

Bromelain seldom causes side effects, but extensive safety studies have not been performed. Allergic reactions may occur in sensitive individuals. Possible side effects include nausea, vomiting, diarrhea, metrorrhagia (bleeding from the uterus, especially at any time other than during the menstrual period), and menorrhagia (excessive bleeding during the menstrual period).[76] Safety is not established in women who are pregnant or breastfeeding.

Other Promising Phytochemicals

Evidence of a cancer-preventive benefit for the following natural compounds is promising, but extremely preliminary. Much more research is necessary.

Blue-Green Algae (Spirulina)

Spirulina is a blue-green algae rich in beta-carotene and other carotenoids. In research conducted by biologist Padmanabhan Nair of the USDA–ARS Beltsville Human Nutrition Research Center in Maryland, a 1-gram spirulina capsule was given daily for a year to 44 tobacco and betel nut chewers in India who had developed precancerous lesions in the mouth (the condition is prevalent in southwestern India). Complete regression of lesions was observed in 20 of 44 (45%) subjects taking the supplement and in only 3 of 43 (7%) taking a placebo (inactive agent). Within 1 year of stopping spirulina, 9 of 20 (45%) complete responders developed recurrent lesions. Spirulina was not associated with toxicity. The researchers said that this was the first human study evaluating the chemopreventive potential of spirulina and that more studies are needed.

Blue-green algae used in supplements comes in over 1,000 different strains that grow in lakes and oceans. The pond variety is the one usually used in supplements. Some algae has been linked to reports of illness and toxicity, possibly due to contamination.

Broccoli (Sulforaphane)

Sulforaphane (also spelled sulphoraphane) is a phytochemical found in broccoli and other members of the Brassica or cruciferous vegetable family such as kale, cauliflower, cabbage, brussels sprouts, and mustard greens.

Though human studies are yet to be done, the rationale for a cancer preventive effect of sulforaphane is compelling. Laboratory studies show the phytochemical is a powerful stimulant of phase 2 enzymes, which block the progression of cancer.[77]

In one study, female rats were fed extracts of broccoli sprouts for 5 days, then exposed along with a control group to a potent carcinogen called DMBA. The extract-fed rats developed fewer tumors and those that got cancers had smaller tumors that took longer to develop. This latest research had its roots in a 1992 experiment which found that sulforaphane added to human cells growing in a lab dish stimulated the cells to increase their production of anticancer phase 2 enzymes.[78] These studies were conducted by Paul Talalay, M.D., director of Johns Hopkins University's Brassica Chemoprotection Laboratory. Talalay has been a long-time advocate of the cancer-fighting benefits of full grown broccoli.[79]

Sulforaphane is much more concentrated in the sprout, which is midway between the dry seed and the green vegetable. Unlike vitamins, manufactured by the plant as it grows, sulforaphane lives in the dormant seed. As the seedling grows, the compound spreads throughout the vegetable. The seeds and 3-day-old sprouts were found to be "extraordinarily high" in the enzyme that neutralizes carcinogens and free radicals. The sprouts, much more edible than the seeds, aren't bitter and don't taste like broccoli, though they possess "a little zing."

When the sprouts are crushed during chewing, they release a chemical that turns into sulforaphane. The longer the plants grow, the more diluted this chemical precursor of sulforaphane becomes—that's why it has to harvested early on. "To get the amount of sulforaphane you find in an ounce or two of sprouts, you'd have to eat about two pounds of broccoli," said Talalay.[80] "Three-day-old broccoli sprouts consistently contain 20 to 50 times the amount of chemoprotective compounds found in mature broccoli heads, and may offer a simple, dietary means of chemically reducing cancer risk," he said.

Talalay is currently studying whether eating a few tablespoonfuls of the sprouts would work. The sprouts resemble alfalfa sprouts and taste similarly to them, he said. Cooking or microwaving does not appear to destroy sulforaphane.[81] Talalay's group is one of the few to do the "very difficult, nitty-gritty studies" of the molecular mechanisms by which diets rich in vegetables inhibit cancer, said Lee W. Wattenberg of the University of Minnesota, who thinks this groundwork may pave the way for turning broccoli extracts into cancer-fighting dietary supplements.

In addition, Talalay envisions that synthetic compounds will be developed to help the body ward off carcinogens, though it will take several years of clinical trials to prove safety and efficacy. "For now," he says, "we may get faster and better impact by looking at dietary means of supplying that protection. Eating more fruits and vegetables has long been associated with reduced cancer risk, so it made sense for us to look at vegetables." Talalay is developing a center to certify that any sprouts ultimately marketed contain high quantities of the sulforaphane precursor. His work is supported in part by the National Cancer Institute, the Cancer Research Foundation of America, and the American Institute for Cancer Research.

Johns Hopkins chemistry professor Gary Posner has already fashioned a synthetic version of sulforaphane that outdid the natural form in lab animals and is easier to produce and more stable.

Marion Nestle, director of New York University's department of nutrition cautioned that sprouts may not supply a range of disease-fighting chemicals. "There's a danger in identifying one particular substance and saying this is it. This is all you need. Sure, broccoli has sulforaphane. But peppers have carotenoids; tomatoes are rich in lycopene; garlic and onions contain allium compounds. All these things protect against cancer. A varied diet of fruits and vegetables may provide as many as 10,000 different substances."

Punctuating this almost universally agreed on point, Wattenberg said, "Any protection is likely due to a combination rather than any single chemical" in foods. Wattenberg, a researcher at the University of Minnesota, is a pioneer in research on enzymes that prevent cancer in animals.

It's known that adult broccoli has its own advantages over sprouts—more folic acid and vitamins A, C, and E, and also more fiber, which helps lower colon cancer risk.

Talalay does not argue against the whole foods approach. "We're talking about adding something new to your diet, not taking anything away," he emphasized.

Grapes (Resveratrol)

Resveratrol is a phytochemical found in at least 72 different plants, including mulberries and peanuts, but grapes are its richest source. Wines also contain the compound, with the highest concentration in red wine, which has been linked to cutting the risk of heart disease and heart attack. The high level of the compound in grape skins is thought to help the plant resist fungal infections.

Resveratrol appears to have antioxidant activity and a comprehensive three-way action against cancer: It blocks carcinogens from inflicting damage, inhibits the development and growth of tumors, and coaxes precancerous cells to revert to normal.[82]

Since resveratrol was only recently identified, no definitive human studies have been done. However, the cancer-preventive effects it shows in the lab and in animals is sure to lead to more research.

Resveratrol was recently discovered by John Pezzuto and his team from the University of Illinois. A study published in the January 10, 1997, issue of *Science* detailed their attempts to track down anticancer substances in readily available foods.[83] After hundreds of tests, the grape came out with the highest marks, inhibiting three different stages of cancer development. "Of all the plants we've tested for cancer chemopreventive activity and all the compounds we've seen, this one has the greatest promise," said Pezzuto.

Resveratrol reduced the number of skin tumors in mice by up to 98%, halted the generation of abnormal cells in cultures of human leukemia cells, and blocked inflammation without causing toxicity. So far, tests have been done only in cell cultures and animals, but Pezzuto has lofty aspirations for this type of work. "My hope is that one day we will be taking a dietary supplement as a cancer preventative, just like many people now take multivitamins," he said.

Other researchers are impressed with the range of activity that resveratrol appears to have against cancer, and some believe that there may be even more powerful agents to be found in fruits and vegetables. Thomas W. Kensler of the Johns Hopkins University School of Public Health said that the resveratrol discovery "provides the scientific underpinnings" for studies that have found health benefits from grapes and wine.

Grapeseed extract is a commercial grape formulation that does not contain resveratrol. The extract consists of a group of flavonoids called proanthocyanidins (or procyanidins) that also appear to offer disease-fighting benefit. Mixtures of these compounds, called PCOs, appear to be stronger antioxidants than vitamins C and E, and may possess a cancer-preventive effect of their own. (For more information on grapeseed, see *The Natural Pharmacist: Your Complete Guide to Herbs.*)

Milk and Dairy Foods (Sphingolipids)

Natural compounds called sphingolipids, found in milk and other dairy foods, were found to inhibit malignant tumors in mice and reduce the number of precancerous lesions that may lead to colon cancer, according to a study published in the October 1996 issue of Cancer Research.[84]

Rosemary

The cooking spice rosemary may help prevent breast cancer in rats, according to a study reported in the May 1996 issue of the *Journal of Nutrition*.[85] Study director John Milner of Pennsylvania State University said the results had profound dietary implications and that they "have found a spice that offers protection against a classic model of breast cancer."

The rats were fed a diet supplemented with 1% rosemary—the same as that found in grocery stores—for 2 weeks, then exposed to DMBA, which is similar to the carcinogens found in cigarette smoke and automobile emissions. The rosemary-fed rats showed a 76% reduction in the number of instances of DMBA binding compared to rats in the control group.

Rosemary appears to work in the initiation phase of cancer, when cells first turn bad. The spice significantly inhibited the binding of DMBA, a chemical known to cause cancer, to the DNA in the mammary cells of the rats. It is believed that this binding process is necessary to jump-start cancer.

Interestingly, the positive anticancer effects of rosemary increased with the amount of dietary fat, which Milner said suggests that "people who eat high-fat diets will actually get the most benefit from rosemary." But the type of fat was a factor: A diet high in saturated fats appeared to weaken the protective action of rosemary, while unsaturated fats showed a positive benefit with rosemary.

Ellagic Acid

Ellagic acid, found in fruits and nuts such as raspberries, strawberries, grapes, apples, walnuts, and pecans may have preventive effects against cancers of the skin, liver, and esophagus, and possibly cancers of the lung and cervix.[86] The compound appears to block promoting enzymes and thus neutralize carcinogens before they can damage DNA. A team of researchers is trying to find out if the compound can do in human patients what it does in lab dish cultures: cut plant tumor formation almost tenfold. The compound is believed to be a natural defense against pests, molds, and other dangers. Ellagic acid levels peak in seeds when the fruits are still green. The levels fall by the time the fruit ripens, when animals eat it and spread the seeds. The research team thinks it may be possible to develop a genetically altered strawberry high in ellagic acid. The compound worked as well as the cancer drug methotrexate in stalling tumor growth in mice.[87]

Apples (Quercetin)

Researchers at Finland's National Public Health Institute found that people who ate the most apples lowered their risk of lung cancer by 58%.[88] Apples contain flavonoids, which have antioxidant activity. The scientists suspect a specific flavonoid called quercetin might be the prime protector, but other of the many compounds found in apples could play a role.

Tangerines (Tangetretin and Nobiletin)

Ingredients in tangerines may help stall the growth of breast cancer cells, according to Canadian researchers.[89] They found that the combination of tangetretin and nobiletin, flavonoids in tangerine, were up to 250 times more potent at inhibiting cancer growth than genistein, a substance found in soy-based foods that has shown preventive effects against breast cancer. The tangerine chemicals appeared to boost the benefit of the breast cancer drug tamoxifen as well. These results should be viewed as preliminary only, especially by women with breast cancer.

White Birch Tree (Betulin)

A derivative of birch tree bark has shown a cancer-blocking effect against melanoma, the deadliest type of skin cancer.[90] Scientists rounded up birch tree bark from a parking lot and extracted betulin from it. From this they synthesized betulinic acid and tested it and other drugs on human cancer cell cultures of melanoma and non-melanoma skin cancers, as well as cancers of the lymph glands, lung, and liver.

Betulinic acid was unique in that it attacked only melanoma cells. "We don't know why," said pharmaceutical biologist John M. Pezzuto in a report in *Nature Medicine*. Most anticancer agents attack a variety of cancers as well as some normal body cells. It seemed that betulinic acid was interacting with something that existed only in melanomas.

When researchers injected human melanoma cells into mice with weakened immune systems, the compound "completely inhibited the growth of tumors," said Pezzuto. Tumor growth in mice with existing melanomas was stifled. However, this does not mean that oral use of white birch will treat melanoma.

Pawpaw Tree Bark

Jerry McLaughlin, a researcher at Purdue University, has found phytochemicals in the bark of the pawpaw tree that seem to be effective in killing even cancer tumors that resist other anticancer agents. The pawpaw tree has the largest fruit native to North America.[91] Again, however, this does not mean that pawpaw bark itself can treat cancer.

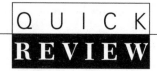

- The evidence is fairly strong that foods high in lycopene (tomatoes and pink grapefruit), isoflavone phytoestrogens such as genistein (soybeans and soy products such as tofu) and lignans (flaxseed oil), polyphenol flavonoids (green tea), and organosulfides (garlic and onion) may help prevent cancer in humans.

Tomatoes and grapefruit: One to two servings a day may be beneficial.

Soy Foods: Typical recommendations for soy foods suggest that one to two servings of soy daily produce a beneficial effect, while concentrated soy isoflavones can be taken at a dose of 40 to 60 mg daily.

Green Tea: The usual serving is 1 to 3 cups daily.

Garlic: A typical recommended dose of garlic is one to two cloves daily. It is not clear whether dried, powdered garlic supplements sold for the purpose of lowering cholesterol have the same effect as whole garlic. Garlic appears to have a blood-thinning effect, and it should not be combined with blood-thinning drugs such as warfarin (Coumadin) or heparin except under the supervision of a physician.

Onion: About $1/4$ cup to 1 cup of chopped onions daily may provide a benefit.

Flaxseed Oil: The typical supplemental dose of flaxseed oil recommended by some nutritionists is 1 to 2 tablespoons daily. Flaxseed oil is easily damaged by heat and light, so don't cook with it. The most palatable way to take it is by adding it to foods, such as using it as a salad dressing.

- There is some evidence that licorice, ginseng, lactobacilli, melatonin, turmeric and curcumin, berberine (goldenseal), and bromelain may be helpful as well. See the chapter for dosage and safety issues.

- Other promising phytochemicals that warrant additional studies include blue-green algae (spirulina), sulforaphane in cruciferous vegetables such as broccoli, resveratrol in grapes, sphingolipids in milk and dairy products, rosemary, ellagic acid in fruits, quercetin in apples, hesperidin and naringin in citrus juices, tangetretin and nobiletin in tangerines, betulin in white birch, and the bark of the pawpaw tree.

Live a Healthful Lifestyle

Diet, of course, is part of living a healthy lifestyle, but it has already grabbed a chapter of its own. Here we'll cover exercise and weight control, smoking, alcohol intake, and other important lifestyle issues.

Exercise and Weight Control: A Foundation for Good Health

You can harvest substantial health benefits just by adding a little exercise to your daily life. A bonus is that exercise helps control weight.

Obesity—usually defined as being 20 to 30% over your ideal weight—appears to increase the risk of endometrial cancer and probably breast cancer in postmenopausal women, and may play a role in other cancers. Numerous studies have linked regular physical activity to a lower risk of certain cancers.[1] Occupational surveys and studies of recreational activity show an association between sedentary (physically inactive) living and the risk of colon cancer, in both men and women. More limited data suggest that physical activity during leisure time is associated with a reduced risk of breast and reproductive system cancers in women. Since moderate exercise elevates mood and helps conserve lean muscle tissue, it may also be beneficial after cancer has been diagnosed.

Add exercise to the benefits of dietary fiber in helping to prevent colon cancer. Women who walked an hour daily reduced their risk of colon cancer by about half. That was the finding from an analysis of the Nurses' Health Study of almost 68,000 women by researchers at Brigham and Women's Hospital and the Harvard School of Public Health.[2] "You don't have to be training for a marathon to get this benefit," said Maria Elena Martinez, an epidemiologist and one of the authors. "These are 50- to 70-year-old women who just get out there and walk." Similar benefits were also found for other types of regular exercise such as biking, jogging, and other aerobic activity for about 30 minutes a day. Studies in men have shown similar results. It is thought that exercise bolsters the immune system, speeds food through the digestive tract so that potential carcinogens spend less time in contact with the colon, and may

Exercise bolsters the immune system and speeds food through the digestive tract so that potential carcinogens spend less time in contact with the colon.

moderate sex hormone levels. Those who exercised the most also tended to have the most favorable lean body weight.

How Much Exercise Do You Need?

When you think of exercise, you may imagine a sweat-drenched body pushing itself to the max in the weight room or on a treadmill. But you don't have to go till you drop, and you don't even have to exercise as "regularly" as you might think to lose weight and help prevent cancer. The current thinking by fitness experts is that less can be more.

If your exercise regimen is too intense or time-consuming, you may not stick with it. Most experts think that the key is to find the type of exercise you enjoy—whether weight-training, aerobics, walking, swimming, or sports activities—and the level of exertion that makes you feel good. It's not the time or intensity—or even frequency, within reason—of exercising that is most important, but the regularity over the long term.[3]

According to aerobics expert Dr. Kenneth H. Cooper, exercising too intensely causes the body to release hazardous free radicals.[4] Lower-intensity exercise may be best because it minimizes the output of free radicals as you work out and beefs up the natural antioxidants in your body at the same time. Cooper thinks that the most effective exercise program

In another study, researchers followed 17,607 men ages 30 to 79 for up to 26 years and assessed their physical activity (self-reported stair climbing, walking, and participation in sports or recreational activities) in relation to cancers of the colon, rectum, lung, prostate, and pancreas.[5] Those most active reduced their risk of colon and lung cancer dramatically—by 44 to 81% for colon cancer and by 38 to 61% for lung cancer. However, there was no signifi-

for good health and build up of defenses against free radical damage is to exercise several times a week at your target heart rate. Maintain that level of exercise at least 30 continuous minutes 3 times a week, or for 20 continuous minutes 4 times a week.

To figure your personal target heart rate, subtract your age from 220—this is your predicted maximal heart rate (heartbeats per minute). Multiply that by 0.65 and then 80% to obtain your target heart rate range. If you are 40 years old, for example, the range you want to stay within during exercise is 117 to 144 heartbeats a minute. Here is how that was figured:

$$220 - 40 = 180$$
$$180 \times 0.65 = 117$$
$$180 \times 0.80 = 144$$

Before starting an exercise program, check with your physician. If you're inexperienced, you may also wish to get advice from an exercise specialist.

cant association between activity and cancers of the rectum, prostate, or pancreas.

In a review of published studies on physical activity and colorectal cancer through March 1997, the authors found a 50% lower risk of colon cancer among people with the highest level of physical activity at work or during leisure time. The findings were adjusted to rule out the effects of diet and other risk factors. The results were not as pronounced for combined colon and rectal cancers.[6]

What to Avoid or Reduce

Part of keeping yourself healthy is knowing what *not* to do. In regard to smoking, the bluntest advice is the best—stop or don't ever start. The advice for alcohol intake, on the other hand, is not so rigid. Here we look at a few "no-no's" and some "maybe so's."

Smoking/Tobacco

Tobacco smoking is the most significant known carcinogen to humans and is the largest single avoidable cause of premature death internationally. Up to 30% of all cancers in developed countries are tobacco-related, with lung cancer being the most prevalent disease linked to smoking.[7]

> **Tobacco smoking is the most significant known carcinogen to humans and is the largest single avoidable cause of premature death internationally.**

Based on an analysis of thirty population studies, passive smoking is now classified as a human lung carcinogen by the U.S. Environmental Protection Agency. Passive smoking causes an estimated 1,500 deaths in nonsmoking women and 500 deaths in nonsmoking men yearly.

Worldwide, the increase in smoking and lung cancer is rising steadily, especially in women. In Japan, lung cancer deaths are ten times higher in men and eight times higher in women since 1950.

During the same time period in China, the increased prevalence of cigarette smoking correlates with a rise in tobacco-related diseases and smoking-related cancers. The situation is similar in central and Eastern Europe.

It's worth repeating: Stop smoking or don't ever start. If you need help quitting, check with a local hospital about available smoking cessation resources. A program might include nicotine replacement therapy and/or the prescription drug bupropion.

The U.S. Environmental Protection Agency now classifies passive smoking as a human lung carcinogen.

Alcohol (Ethanol)

Alcohol intake—drinking wine, beer, or liquor—is strongly associated with the risk of dying from cancers of the mouth, pharynx, esophagus, and larynx. Drinking combined with smoking greatly increases the risk. Additionally, the death rate from breast cancer was 30% higher among women who consumed at least one drink daily.[8, 9] These were the findings from the huge Cancer Prevention Study II, in which 490,000 people were followed for 9 years. Researchers adjusted for smoking and other risk factors to rule out their effects on the results. The amount of alcohol consumed is important. Generally, cancer risk begins to climb with as few as two drinks a day. The risk is 3 to 7 times higher among both men and women with at least four drinks a day. A drink is defined as 12 ounces of beer, 5 ounces of wine, or 1.5 ounces of 80-proof liquor. Breast, colorectal, liver, and pancreatic cancers also have been linked to alcohol intake.

Though the American Cancer Society discourages alcohol use, it acknowledges that moderate intake—two

Nell's Story

The doctor told Nell, 53, that her high blood pressure was under good control and to keep taking the same dose of her medication. "Have you had any luck in trying to quit smoking?" he asked.

"I know I said I'd try to stop," she said, "and I do intend to quit soon—maybe when the stress at work lets up." She understood that smoking was a huge risk factor for heart disease, which was their main concern.

"When we talked about it last time," the doctor said, reading his notes, "you mentioned that you also drink a cocktail or glass of wine most evenings."

"Yes, that's good for my heart, isn't it?"

"Ordinarily it might be," he said. "But it's a fine line. When you go beyond that line in alcohol intake," he added, "you in-

drinks a day for men and one for women—appears to lower the risk of heart disease in middle-aged adults, and that this benefit may outweigh its cancer risk in men over age 50 and women over age 60. However, women at unusually high risk for breast cancer may wish to consider abstaining from alcohol.

Alcohol intake is strongly associated with cancers of the mouth, pharynx, esophagus, larynx, and breast.

Excessive Sun Exposure

There is little doubt that getting too much sun exposure can cause skin damage and increase the chances of skin cancer. Beyond that, the risk versus bene-

crease your risk of cancer. If you were at high risk for breast cancer I would advise you not to drink at all."

Smoking, he emphasized, was the real problem in her case. Not only was smoking a major cancer risk factor by itself, it greatly amplified the cancer-promoting effects of alcohol. The combination was a "double whammy" for cancer, as he put it.

That was a real eye-opener for her. She realized that quitting smoking, as tough as it might be, was the best thing she could do to gain control of her health. As a first step, Nell agreed to make an appointment for smoking cessation counseling.

fits of sun exposure is a hot debate. It is thought that appropriate amounts of sun may have a preventive effect against breast cancer and some other cancers due to the protective effect of sun-induced vitamin D production.

A paper titled "Sunlight—Can It Prevent as Well as Cause Cancer?" first published in 1995 in the journal *Cancer Research* suggested that the benefits of regular sunlight exposure may outweigh its skin cancer risks.[10] Sun exposure is thought to play a preventive role in breast, ovarian, colon, and prostate cancer. A 1993 study estimated that regular tanning might prevent 30,000 of the 138,000 Americans who die from these cancers yearly. The reasoning is that far fewer people die from sunburn-related skin cancers than the other forms of cancer, and most skin cancer deaths can be prevented when the disease is detected early. Coauthor George P. Studzinski of the UMD–New Jersey Medical School in Newark said that encouraging people to avoid sun exposure may be denying them the anticancer benefits of sunlight and that regular, moderate sun exposure should be encouraged. But not everyone agrees.

"The major point is that there is nothing healthy about a tan," said an American Cancer Society spokesperson. "A tan is how the body attempts to protect itself against damage from the sun."

If you do decide to avoid exposing your skin to the sun, keep in mind that there is considerable debate about the reliability of a sunscreen to protect fair-skinned individuals from the sun's harmful rays.[11] "It's not safe to rely on sunscreen," said Marianne Berwick of the Memorial Sloan-Kettering Cancer Center in New York. There is convincing evidence, she thinks, that using a sunscreen may not prevent skin cancer, particularly the most dangerous form—melanoma.

There is debate about whether using a sunscreen can prevent skin cancer, particularly the most dangerous form— melanoma.

At one time, the most dangerous form of ultraviolet radiation from the sun was thought to be UV-B, and the first sunscreen products blocked only UV-B radiation. Then scientists studied the UV-A rays generated at tanning salons and found that UV-A may cause more long-term damage than UV-B. Some products claiming both UV-B and UV-A protection contain chemicals that absorb some UV-A light, but their main efficacy lies in the traditional UV-B range, bringing into question their strength as UV-A blockers. Zinc oxide and titanium dioxide completely block all forms of UV radiation, but they produce an unsightly white coating. Newer formulations of titanium dioxide–containing products may be more cosmetically acceptable.

A conservative view held by many skin experts is that sunscreens should be used year-round, not just in the summer months, especially by people who are avid golfers, or athletes who train during winter months and get a fair amount of sun exposure.

"A lot of evidence suggests that damage occurs before the point of redness," said Mark Naylor, M.D., a dermatologist at the University of Oklahoma. "So I do not believe that SPF 15 is the highest you will ever need, especially for anyone who has had skin cancer or is fair-skinned, because they would need an SPF 30 or higher." (SPF refers to Sun Protection Factor; the higher the number, the greater the protection.)

He also stressed the need to reapply sunscreen throughout the day because many people don't apply it often enough for continuous protection. "Children benefit the most from sunscreens, more so than adults," Naylor continued, "because early life sunburns and overexposures are closely linked to skin cancer." He said that children should receive at least the same level of sunscreen as adults, "or an even higher SPF to make sure they do not get burned."

Here are the American Medical Association's 10 Sun Safety Guidelines for Children and Parents:

1. Keep infants out of the sun—especially those under 6 months of age.
2. Avoid sun exposure from 10 A.M. to 3 P.M.
3. Use a sunscreen—one that is perspiration and water-resistant—with an SPF of at least 15.

4. For infants and toddlers, use carriages with a hood attachment or attach an umbrella; provide wide-brimmed hats to shield young children from harmful rays and light-colored clothing to reflect the sun.

5. Beware of reflected light around water, as well as cloudy days—as much as 80% of the sun's radiation passes through clouds.

6. Be cautious of photosensitivity with certain medications, such as tetracycline (ask your pharmacist about your medications).

7. Make sure lenses of sunglasses absorb 100% of UV-A and UV-B light, and encourage children to wear safe sunglasses to possibly prevent or delay eye problems later in life.

8. Avoid tanning parlors.

9. Examine skin regularly—early detection of skin cancer is critical. Look for unusual growths, itchy patches, changes in moles or colored areas.

10. Set a good example for your children by applying these same rules to yourself. And don't forget to cover the vulnerable areas often overlooked—the lips and ears.

Skin cancers associated with UV radiation from the sun are the most common form of cancer. Despite suggestions that sunscreens may not afford as much protection as once thought, these products are the best protection—other than clothing—you've got against skin cancer.

Viral Infections

There is strong evidence that viral infections increase the risk for several cancers.[12] Human papilloma virus is associated with an increased risk of cervical cancer, Epstein-Barr virus with nasopharyngeal cancer, hepatitis B virus with primary liver cancer, and HIV with Kaposi's sarcoma and some forms of lymphoma. All totaled, viral-related cancers represent about 11% of all cancers worldwide. Vaccinations against such viral infections could have a considerable positive impact, especially in developing countries, where infection rates are higher.

Radon

Radon is a naturally occurring odorless and colorless radioactive gas found in most homes. As radon decays, it releases radioactive particles that can damage lung cells.[13] It is harmless when dispersed in the air, but can be toxic when improper ventilation allows it to build up inside—that is one potential drawback to having an air-tight, "energy-saving" home. The EPA estimates that about one in fifteen homes may have excessive levels. Radon is the second leading cause of lung cancer in the United States (behind cigarette smoking), and may contribute to as many as 20,000 cancer deaths yearly.

The gas seeps into the home from the soil through the foundations. Many countries have new building regulations that require all new homes to be fitted with anti-radon devices, such as mechanical underfloor ventilation, to reduce concentrations of the gas. Radon test kits are widely available to those wishing to check their home for possible high radon levels.

A recent British study found that residential radon gas and smoking are an additive lethal combination. Richard Doll, a consultant with the Imperial Cancer Research Fund Clinical Trial Service Unit, said that radon and smoking interact with each other to multiply the risk of getting lung cancer. In a news release, he said that "most radon-induced lung cancers are produced in conjunction with cigarette smoking and, in the absence of smoking, the number produced would be much smaller."

Undeserved Bad Raps

Concern about cancer can cause much worry about possible carcinogens we're exposed to in our daily lives. Here we look at some things which may have unjustified fears attached to them.

Food Irradiation, Salt, Coffee, Fluoride

According to the American Cancer Society, there is no evidence that irradiation of foods, dietary salt, coffee, or fluoride increase cancer risk. Irradiation of foods is used to kill harmful bacteria and does not remain in foods after treatment.

According to the American Cancer Society, there is no evidence that irradiation of foods, dietary salt, coffee, or fluoride increase cancer risk.

There is little evidence that moderate amounts of salt or salt-preserved foods affect cancer risk. However, some evidence suggests that diets containing large amounts of foods preserved by salting and pickling may be related to an increased risk for cancers of the stomach, nose, and throat.

The most recent scientific studies have found no link between coffee and the risk of cancer of the pancreas, breast, or any other cancers. Caffeine may increase symptoms of fibrocystic breast lumps in some women, and this fact has led to media articles about coffee in relation to breast cancer.

Extensive research that examined the use of fluorides in dental treatment, toothpaste, public water supplies, and foods found that fluorides do not increase cancer risk.

Electromagnetic Fields

Despite two decades of concern and debate, electromagnetic fields from electrical power lines apparently don't cause cancer, according to a major study published in the *New England Journal of Medicine.* The study was supported by the National Cancer Institute and the University of Minnesota Children's Cancer Research Fund. It confirms the conclusions released previously by the National Research Council.[14]

Hair Dye

The rising incidence of breast cancer and the fact that about one-third of American women use permanent hair dyes has raised concern about the potential for hair dyes to act as mutagens or carcinogens that may lead to cancer in humans. However, a large American Cancer Society study reported in the *Journal of the National Cancer Institute* showed that hair dyes do not increase cancer deaths, even in those using them for 20 years or more, with the possible exception of black hair dye.[15] The study involved over half a million women followed for more than 6 years. Even long durations of use of hair dyes did not increase the risk of breast, digestive system, genital, hematopoietic (leukemia, lymphoma), or brain cancers. Prior studies had also shown no strong association. The possible increased risk of lung cancer in the current study was nullified when researchers took cigarette smoking into account.

However, there was an increased risk for developing non-Hodgkin's lymphoma or multiple myeloma in women who used black hair dye over a prolonged time period. Earlier studies had found a higher risk with darker colors of permanent hair dye such as black, brown, and red. In light of the current study results, it may be prudent for women not to use black hair dyes for prolonged periods.

An editorial said that the evidence for cancer risk was not sufficient to avoid hair dye use.

Stress and Cancer

Much of what we know in this area concerns how stress affects the immune system. However, the role of the immune system in cancer is still not clear, and no one can say whether the types of immune changes induced by stress are important in cancer.

There is substantial evidence that psychological stress can alter immune function, according to an editorial in the January 7, 1998, *Journal of the National Cancer Institute* written by Carnegie Mellon psychologist Sheldon Cohen and University of Pittsburgh Medical School immunologist Bruce Rabin.[16]

There are a number of biologic pathways by which stress could impact immune function, they said, including nerves that connect the brain and immune system, and stress-caused release of hormones from the brain that influence immune cells. Stress might also alter immunity an additional way through its effects on behaviors such as increases in smoking, drinking alcohol, and loss of sleep.

There is substantial evidence that psychological stress can alter immune function.

Anxiety about having cancer might itself undermine your body's strength to battle the disease. Unlike many other diseases, cancer often makes the patient feel his or her body is a traitor as cancer cells strike out to claim areas made up of normal cells. The patient may feel diseased as a person, rather than just having a diseased body part. This change in view of the self creates additional stress.[17]

Researchers at Ohio State University Medical Center used a standard questionnaire to measure stress levels in 116 women after they had breast cancer surgery but before they started chemotherapy. The women who felt most overwhelmed by their diagnosis and treatment showed inhibited immune responses reflected in natural killer cell and T-cell responses. (Killer cells are sent out by the immune system to find and destroy invading cells.)[18]

That doesn't necessarily mean that worrying causes cancer, said virologist Ronald Glaser, one of the study researchers. The significance of the role played by killer cells in relation to cancer is not known.

But these results may add another peg to findings of previous studies showing that breast cancer and malignant melanoma patients who joined a support group lived longer.[19] Support groups help people manage both the disease and the fears associated with it, and complement the support of partners and loved ones. Government health officials have acknowledged the importance of breast cancer support groups for women in the military services and are establishing such groups for both patients and families.[20]

Current trials are underway to find out if counseling and support groups can enhance killer cell activity and if doing that might raise the odds of beating cancer.

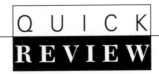

QUICK REVIEW

- Exercise and weight control are prime ways to lower your cancer risk and enjoy good health in general. You don't need to exercise strenuously to get protective benefits—regular exercise over the long term may be more important than the time or frequency you put in.

- Environmental exposures known to increase your cancer risk include smoking, excessive ultraviolet light from the sun or tanning parlors, certain viruses, and radon. There is little evidence that electromagnetic fields, hair dyes (except black), food irradiation, salt, coffee, or fluoride increase cancer risk.

- Stopping smoking would reduce about 30% of all cancer cases. Even passive smoking is risky.

- More than very moderate regular ingestion of alcoholic beverages can increase cancer risk, especially when combined with smoking.

- Sun exposure is a mixed bag. Brief periods in the sun may confer a protective effect against several cancers (presumably due to the stimulation of vitamin D production), but too much sun exposure is associated with skin cancer.

- Studies suggest that cancer patients who join a support group may live longer, and research is underway to find out more.

Putting It All Together

For your easy reference this chapter contains a brief summary of key information contained in this book. Please refer to earlier chapters for more comprehensive information, including a detailed discussion of safety issues.

Now that you've read this book, the road to natural cancer prevention should be clear: The best way to prevent cancer is to live a healthful lifestyle. It's also wise to assess your cancer risk and use preventive screenings.

A healthful lifestyle includes eating a balanced diet of whole foods, using appropriate nutritional supplements in reasonable amounts for extra protection, avoiding smoking, watching your alcohol consumption, and making sure you get enough exercise.

Assess Your Cancer Risk and Use Preventive Screenings

Know your cancer risk factors (see chapter 2). That helps you determine which screening tests should be done to catch any potential cancer early, when it is most likely to be curable (see chapter 3).

Be aware of the seven *general* warning symptoms of cancer. CAUTION is an acronym derived by combining the first letters of each item:

Change in bowel or bladder habits.
A sore that doesn't heal.
Unusual bleeding or discharge.
Thickening or lump in breast or elsewhere.
Indigestion or difficulty in swallowing.
Obvious change in wart or mole.
Nagging cough or hoarseness.

Eat an Anticancer Diet

At least 30% of cancers are related to diet. Numerous studies show that your best protection against cancer is to eat a primarily plant-based diet with a variety of fresh fruits and vegetables and whole grains. The USDA's Nutrition Facts food label and food guide pyramid are valuable tools that make it easier than ever before to select health-smart foods (see chapter 4).

In addition to providing a bevy of cancer-preventive nutrients and phytochemicals, such a diet is low in fat and high in fiber and also protects against heart disease and other chronic diseases. The key to this protection may be the way the natural substances in whole foods work together. You can significantly lower your cancer risk by regularly eating certain foods and avoiding others.

Limit the amount of fat (especially saturated or animal fat) in your diet and favor white meats (chicken and fish) over red meats (beef, pork, and lamb). Dry beans (such as pinto, navy, kidney, and black beans) can serve as meat alternatives. Dietary fats may be associated with an increased risk of cancers of the breast, ovary, prostate, colon, and lung. Red meat has also been linked to several cancers, particularly colon and prostate cancer, and possibly breast and pancreatic cancer. Monounsaturated fats such as olive oil and canola oil may actually have a protective effect against breast cancer and possibly other cancers. Reduce total fat in your diet to below 30% of daily calories.

Avoid or reduce your consumption of pickled and salt-cured meats. Avoid eating overcooked or charred foods. Grilling and excessive cooking of meats produces cancer-causing compounds, and frequent eating of grilled or barbecued meats may increase the chances of getting cancer of the stomach or esophagus. Safer cooking methods include baking, roasting, and broiling.

Natural Treatments That May Reduce Your Cancer Risk

Certain nutritional supplements may provide extra insurance against cancer (see chapter 5). **Vitamins C, E, beta-carotene,** and the mineral **selenium** are antioxidants, agents that can neutralize free radicals, which are toxic compounds that can damage DNA and jumpstart cancer. Foods high in antioxidant nutrients exert a significant cancer-preventive effect.

Among supplemental nutrients, vitamin E, selenium, and multivitamin formulations have the best evidence backing them as cancer preventives.

Vitamin E in supplement form appears to significantly lower the risk of prostate cancer, as well as to protect against cancers of the colon, mouth, and throat. Foods high in vitamin E protect against cancers of the colon, stomach, mouth, throat, esophagus, liver, and breast (hereditary).

Selenium in supplement form appears to lower the risk of cancers of the prostate, colon, rectum, and lung, as well as reduce cancer deaths by 50%. Foods high in selenium are associated with a lower risk for cancers of the esophagus and stomach.

Multivitamin formulations appear to substantially cut the risk of colon cancer, as well as provide a host of vitamins that may be protective in other ways. Foods rich in beta-carotene protect against several cancers, but there is currently no meaningful evidence that supplemental beta-carotene offers significant protection against cancer, and evidence suggests that it may actually be harmful, at least in smokers and asbestos workers. Beta-carotene needs can easily be met through the diet, and it may be best to get it this way until more is known.

Vitamin C–rich foods exert cancer-preventive effects, but so far there is no convincing evidence that vitamin C in supplement form protects against cancer.

Dietary **folic acid** may protect against colorectal and cervical cancers, but it is not known whether supplementary folic acid confers the same benefit. Folic acid supplementation may be able to help reverse cervical dysplasia in women taking oral contraceptives, but a doctor's supervision is mandatory.

The evidence is minimal and less persuasive for vitamin D, molybdenum, and calcium.

The antioxidant nutrients appear to work together to enhance overall benefit. A reasonable daily regimen of nutritional supplementation might include a comprehensive multivitamin–mineral formulation, vitamin E (100 to 400 IU), selenium (50 to 200 mcg), and vitamin C (at least 200 mg).

Additionally, supplemental herbs or food phytochemicals may firm up your supplements' insurance policy, especially if you don't eat a balanced diet (see chapter 6). In test tube studies, phytochemicals have been found to stall or reverse almost every step in the development of cancer. Some human studies have been done, but there is still much we don't know. In studies of whole foods, the strongest cancer preventives so far identified appear to be lycopene (tomatoes and pink grapefruit), isoflavone phytoestrogens such as genistein (soybeans and soy products such as tofu) and lignans (flaxseed oil), polyphenol flavonoids (green tea), organosulfides (garlic and onion), and possibly sulforaphane (cruciferous vegetables such as broccoli, kale, cauliflower, cabbage, brussels sprouts, and mustard greens). These compounds are generally available in supplement form. You can also find concentrated whole-food supplements such as cruciferous vegetables (broccoli, cabbage, cauliflower, and so on) in extract or freeze-dried form in capsules, tablets, and powder. Whole-food supplements might come closest to matching the beneficial effects seen in the dietary studies.

Live a Healthful Lifestyle

Besides eating a healthful diet, living a healthful lifestyle means avoiding smoking, exercising regularly, limiting the consumption of alcoholic beverages, using caution in sexual activity, and getting a regular medical checkup (see chapter 7).

1. About 30% of cancers are linked to smoking. The best advice is the bluntest: Don't smoke. That's easier said than done, but the damaging impact of this one risk factor (both active and passive smoking) is so great on you and your family that it's worth every effort to stop smoking or never start.

2. Exercise a minimum of 3 times a week for at least 30 minutes per session to control weight and promote overall health. Regular physical activity is associated with a lower risk of colon and lung cancer. Obesity may increase the risk of endometrial and breast cancer as well as other chronic diseases such as diabetes and heart disease.

3. Consume alcoholic beverages in moderation if at all. Men should limit their intake to less than two drinks

daily and women to one drink daily. The combination of alcohol and smoking is especially harmful, further increasing the risk of cancer of the oral cavity, pharynx, esophagus, and larynx. Additionally, breast, colorectal, liver, and pancreatic cancer have been linked to alcohol intake. Two drinks a day for men and one for women appears to lower the risk of heart disease in middle-aged adults, and this benefit may outweigh its cancer risk in men over age 50 and women over age 60. However, women at unusually high risk for breast cancer may wish to consider abstaining from alcohol.

4. Be cautious in sexual activity. Use a condom to protect yourself from possible exposure to viral infections such as the human papilloma virus and hepatitis B virus, which are linked to an increased risk of cervical cancer and primary liver cancer, respectively. A vaccination is available for the hepatitis B virus.

5. Get an annual health checkup, especially if you are over 40. Medical problems are often discovered during such a routine medical exam.

Notes

Introduction

1. Longo D. Approach to the patient with cancer (ch. 81). *Harrison's Principles of Internal Medicine* 14/e. CD-ROM. New York: McGraw-Hill, 1998.
2. Welland D. 15 cancer-preventing strategies that stack the odds in your favor. Environmental Nutrition 21(3): 1, 1998.

Chapter One

1. Longo D, 1998.
2. Parker SL, et al. Cancer statistics. *Cancer J Clin* 46(1): 5–27, 1996.
3. American Heart Association, American Cancer Society. Living well, staying well. New York: Times Books and Random House, 11, 1996.
4. Osborne M, et al. Cancer prevention. *Lancet* 349 (Suppl 2): SII27–SII30, 1997.
5. Brawley OW and Kramer BS. Prevention and early detection of cancer (ch. 82). *Harrison's Principles of Internal Medicine* 14/e. CD-ROM. New York: McGraw-Hill, 1998; Scott RE, et al. Mechanisms for initiation and promotion of carcinogenesis: a review and a new concept. *Mayo Clinic Proceedings* 59: 107–117, 1984.
6. Jaret P. Closing in on cancer. *Health* 12: 2, 66–77, 1998.

Chapter Two

1. American Cancer Society. Cancer Facts & Figures—1998; http://www.cancer.org/frames.html.

Chapter Three

1. American Cancer Society, 1998.
2. Kaura SK. A family doctor's guide to understanding & preventing cancer. Santa Fe: Healthpress, 229–236, 1991.
3. Jaret P. Truth, beauty, and skin cancer. *Health* 11: 5, 78–85, 1997.
4. Berwick M, et al. Melanoma epidemiology. *Curr Opin Oncol* 9(2): 178–182, 1997.

Chapter Four

1. Key KK and DeNoon DJ. Wheat bran cereals reduce risk of colon cancer. *Cancer Researcher Weekly* 13, October 24, 1994.

2. Nixon DW. The cancer recovery eating plan.. New York and Canada: Times Books and Random House, 1996.

3. Dreher H. Your defense against cancer. New York: Harper & Row, 100–104, 1988.

4. Lichtenstein AH, et al. Dietary fat consumption and health. *Nutr Rev* 56 (5 Pt 2): S3–S19, 1998.

5. Eastman P. Dietary fat manipulations to lower cancer risk are under close scrutiny. *Journal of the National Cancer Institute* 88: 19, 1339–1340, 1996.

6. Lichtenstein AH, et al. Dietary fat consumption and health. *Nutr Rev* 56 (5 Pt 2): S3–S19, 1998; Gaziano JM and Hennekens CH. Dietary fat and risk of prostate cancer. *Journal of the National Cancer Institute* 87: 19, 1427–1428, 1995; Singh J, Hamid R, and Reddy BS. Dietary fat and colon cancer: modulating effect of types and amount of dietary fat on ras-p21 function during promotion and progression stages of colon cancer. *Cancer Research* 57(2): 253–258, 1997.

7. Risch HA, et al. Dietary fat intake and risk of epithelial ovarian cancer. *Journal of the National Cancer Institute* 86(18): 1409–1415, 1994.

8. Alavanja MC, et al. Saturated fat intake and lung cancer risk among nonsmoking women in Missouri. *Journal of the National Cancer Institute* 85(23): 1906–1916, 1993.

9. Willett WC. Specific fatty acids and risks of breast and prostate cancer: dietary intake. *Am J Clin Nutr* 66 (6 Suppl): 1557S–1563S, 1997.

10. Osborne M, et al., 1997.

11. Wynder EL and Cohen LA. Breast cancer: weighing the evidence for a promoting role of dietary fat. *Journal of the National Cancer Institute* 89: 11, 766–775, 1997.

12. Giovannucci E, et al. A prospective study of dietary fat and risk of prostate cancer. *Journal of the National Cancer Institute* 85(19): 1571–1579, 1993.

13. Willett WC, et al. Relation of meat, fat, and fiber intake to the risk of colon cancer in a prospective study among women. *N Engl J Med* 323(24): 1664–1672, 1990.

14. Ward MH, et al. Risk of adenocarcinoma of the stomach and esophagus with meat cooking method and doneness preference. *Int J Cancer* 71(1): 14–19, 1997.

15. Chicken marinade may help prevent cancer. *Tufts University Health & Nutrition Letter* 15: 6, 8, August 1997.

16. Kaura SK, 127, 1991.

17. Welland D, 1998.

18. Hotchkiss JH. Food safety, cancer, and the Delaney Clause. *World & I* 8: 10, 214–221, 1993.
19. Key KK and DeNoon DJ. Scientists discover cancer fighter. *Cancer Researcher Weekly* 12–13, October 3, 1994.
20. Osborne M, et al., 1997.
21. Wolk A, et al. A prospective study of association of monounsaturated fat and other types of fat with risk of breast cancer. *Arch Intern Med.* 158 (1): 41–45, 1998; Jaret, P. Fats to eat, fats to avoid. *Health* 12: 3, 24, April 1998.
22. Wolk A, et al., 1998.
23. Kritchevsky D. Dietary fibre and cancer. *Eur J Cancer Prev* 6 (5): 435–441, 1997; Liebman B. Fiber. *Nutrition Action Health Letter* 21: 7, 1–4, September 1994.
24. Fuchs CS, et al. Dietary fiber and the risk of colorectal cancer and adenoma in women. *N Engl J Med* 340: 169–176, 1999.
25. Marion M. The vegetable hater's guide to nutrition. *Men's Health* 72–76, March 1998.
26. Cooper KH. Dr. Kenneth H. Cooper's antioxidant revolution. Nashville: Thomas Nelson Publishers, 153, 1994.
27. Marion M, 1998.

Chapter Five

1. Key SW and Marble M. Vitamin E, antioxidant nutrients may fight cancer. *Cancer Weekly Plus* 20–21, April 28, 1997.
2. Gey KF, Vitamins E plus C and interacting co-nutrients required for optimal health. A critical and constructive review of epidemiology and supplementation data regarding cardiovascular disease and cancer. *Biofactors* 7 (1–2): 113–174, 1998.
3. Covington R. (Ed.), Handbook of nonprescription drugs. American Pharmaceutical Association, 1996.
4. Gey KF, 1998.
5. Key SW and Marble M, 1997.
6. Knekt P, et al. Vitamin E and cancer prevention. *Am J Clin Nutr* 53 (1 Suppl): 283S–286S, 1991.
7. Losonczy KG, Harris TB, and Havlik RJ. Vitamin E and vitamin C supplement use and risk of all-cause and coronary heart disease mortality in older persons: the Established Populations for Epidemiologic Studies of the Elderly. *Am J Clin Nutr* 64: 190–196, 1996.
8. Heinonen OP, et al. Prostate cancer and supplementation with alpha-tocopherol and beta-carotene: incidence and mortality in a controlled trial. *Journal National Cancer Institute* 90(6): 440–446, 1998.

9. White E, et al. Relationship between vitamin and calcium supplement use and colon cancer. *Cancer Epidemiol Biomarkers Prev* 6(10): 769–774, 1997; Macready N. Vitamins associated with lower colon-cancer risk. *Lancet* 350: 9089, 1452, 1997.

10. Bostick RM, et al. Reduced risk of colon cancer with high intake of vitamin E: the Iowa Women's Health Study. *Cancer Res* 53 (18): 4230–4237, 1993; Colon cancer & vitamin E. *Presidents & Prime Ministers* 3:3, 44, May/June 1994.

11. Gridley G, et al. Vitamin supplement use and reduced risk of oral and pharyngeal cancer. *Am J Epidemiol* 135 (10): 1083–1092, 1992.

12. Zheng W, Sellers TA, Doyle TJ, et al. Retinol, antioxidant vitamins, and cancer of the upper digestive tract in a prospective cohort study of postmenopausal women. *Am J Epidemiol* 142: 955–960, 1995.

13. Ambrosone CB, et al. Interaction of family history of breast cancer and dietary antioxidants with breast cancer risk. (New York, United States). *Cancer Causes Control* 6 (5): 407–15, 1995.

14. Rimm EB and Stampfer MJ. The role of antioxidants in preventive cardiology. *Curr Opin Cardiol* 12 (2): 188–194, 1997.

15. Kiyose C, et al. Biodiscrimination of alpha-tocopherol stereoisomers in humans after oral administration. *Am J Clin Nutr* 65 (3): 785–789, 1997.

16. Burton GW, et al. Human plasma and tissue alpha-tocopherol concentrations in response to supplementation with deuterated natural and synthetic vitamin E. *Am J Clin Nutr* 67 (4): 669–684, 1998.

17. Christen S, et al. Gamma-tocopherol traps mutagenic electrophiles such as NOX and complements alpha-tocopherol: physiological implications. *Proc Natl Acad Sci USA* 94: 3217–3222, 1997.

18. Longo D, Heywood R, et al. Part five—nutrition; the toxicity of beta-carotene. *Toxicology* 36, 91–100, 1985.

19. Longo D, Heywood R, et al., 1985.

20. Covington R. (Ed.) 1996.

21. Covington R. (Ed.) 1996.

22. National Research Council, Diet and Health. 1989. Implications for reducing chronic disease risk. Washington, DC: National Academy Press, 376–379.

23. Clark LC, et al. Effects of selenium supplementation for cancer prevention in patients with carcinoma of the skin. A randomized controlled trial. Nutritional Prevention of Cancer Study Group. *JAMA* 276 (24): 1957–1963, 1996; Selenium may prevent some cancers in patients with history of skin cancer. *Geriatrics* 52 (2): 20, February 1997.

24. Garland M, et al. Prospective study of toenail selenium levels and cancer among women. *Journal of the National Cancer Institute* 276 (7): 497–505, 1995.

25. van den Brandt PA, et al. Toenail selenium levels and the risk of breast cancer. *Am J Epidemiol* 276 (1): 20–26, 1994.

26. Covington R. (Ed.) 387, 1996.

27. Ip C and Lisk DJ. Enrichment of selenium in allium vegetables for cancer prevention. *Carcinogenesis* 276 (9): 1881–1885, 1994; Lavender OA, et al. Bioavailability of selenium to Finnish men as assessed by platelet glutathione peroxidase activity and other blood parameters. *Am J Clin Med* 37, 887–897, 1993; Mutanen M. Biovailability of selenium. *Annals Clin Res* 18, 48–54, 1986; Thomson CD, et al. Effect of prolonged supplementation with daily supplements of selenomethionine and sodium selenite on glutathione peroxidase activity in blood of New Zealand residents. *Am J Clin Nutr* 36, 24–31, 1982.

28. Murray MT. Encyclopedia of nutritional supplements. Prima Publishing, 222, 1996.

29. Fan AM, et al. Selenium: nutritional, toxicological and clinical aspects. *West J Med* 153, 160–167, 1990.

30. Covington R. (Ed.) 366–368, 1996.

31. Steinmetz KA, Potter JD. Vegetables, fruit, and cancer prevention: a review. *J Am Diet Assoc* 96 (10): 1027–1039, 1996.

32. Santamaria L and Bianchi–Santamaria A. Carotenoids in cancer chemoprevention and therapeutic interventions. *J Nutr Sci Vitaminol* (Tokyo) Spec No: 321–326, 1992.

33. Omenn GS, Goodman GE, Thornquist MD, et al. Effects of a combination of beta-carotene and vitamin A on lung cancer and cardiovascular disease. *N Engl J Med* 334:1150–1155, 1996.

34. Hennekens CH, Buring JE, Manson JAE, et al. Lack of effect of long-term supplementation with beta carotene on the incidence of malignant neoplasms and cardiovascular disease. *N Engl J Med* 334 (1996) (18): 1145–1149.

35. Albanes D, Heinonen OP, et al. Alpha-tocopherol and beta-carotene supplements and lung cancer incidence in the alpha-tocopherol, beta-carotene cancer prevention study: effects of base-line characteristics and study compliance. *Journal National Cancer Institute* 88 (21): 1560–1570, 1996.

36. Heinonen OP, et al., 1998.

37. The trials of beta-carotene: Is the verdict in? *Tufts University Diet & Nutrition Letter* 14: 1, 4–6, 1996.

38. Kohlmeier L and Hastings SB. Epidemiologic evidence of a role of carotenoids in cardiovascular disease prevention. *Am J Clin Nutr* 62 (Suppl): 1370S–1376S, 1995.

39. White WS, et al. Pharmacokinetics of beta-carotene and canthaxanthin after individual and combined doses by human subjects. *J Am Coll Nutr* 13: 665–671, 1994.

40. Toma S, et al. Treatment of oral leukoplakia with beta-carotene. *Oncology* 49, 77–81, 1992.

41. Muto Y, et al. Growth retardation in human cervical dysplasia–derived cell lines by beta-carotene through down-regulation of epidermal growth factor receptor. *Am J Clin Nutr* 62 (6 Suppl): 1535S–1540S, 1995.

42. Giuliano AR and Gapstur S. Can cervical dysplasia and cancer be prevented with nutrients? *Nutr Rev* 56 (1 Pt 1): 9–16, 1998.

43. Marble M and Key SW. WHO: Carotenoid pills should not be promoted. *Cancer Weekly Plus* 16–23, February 1998.

44. Cooper KH, 148, 1994.

45. Longo D, Heywood R, et al., 1985.

46. Key SW. Researchers say more to story of beta-carotene and cancer. *Cancer Biotechnology Weekly* 11–12, February 5–12, 1996.

47. Gey KF, 113–174, 1998.

48. Head KA. Ascorbic acid in the prevention and treatment of cancer. *Altern Med Rev* 3 (3): 174–186, 1998.

49. Head KA., 1998; Shibata A, et al. Intake of vegetables, fruits, beta-carotene, Vitamin C and vitamin supplements and cancer incidence among the elderly: a prospective study. *Br J Cancer* 66 (4): 673–679, 1992; Cohen M and Bhagavan HN. Ascorbic acid and gastrointestinal cancer. *J Am Coll Nutr* 14 (6): 565–578, 1995; Esteve J, et al. Diet and cancers of the larynx and hypopharynx: the IARC multi-center study in southwestern Europe. *Cancer Causes Control* 7: 240–252, 1996; Flagg EW, et al. Epidemiologic studies of antioxidants and cancer. *J Am Coll Nutr* 1495: 419–427, 1995; Block G. Epidemiologic evidence regarding vitamin C and cancer. *Am J Clin Nutr* 54: 1310S–1314S, 1991.

50. Daviglus ML, et al. Dietary beta-carotene, vitamin C, and risk of prostate cancer: results from the Western Electric study. *Epidemiology* 7 (5): 472–477, 1996.

51. Block G. Vitamin C and cancer prevention: the epidemiologic evidence. *Am J Clin Nutr* 53 (1 Suppl): 270S–282S, 1991.

52. Cohen M, Bhagavan, HN. Ascorbic acid and gastrointestinal cancer. *J Am Coll Nutr* 14 (6): 565–578, 1995; Ocke M, Kromhout D, Menotti A, et al. Average intake of antioxidant (pro) vitamins and subsequent cancer mortality in the 16 cohorts of the seven countries study. *Int J Cancer* 61(4): 480–484, 1995.

53. Bruemmer B, et al. Nutrient intake in relation to bladder cancer among middle-aged men and women. *Am J Epidemiol* 144 (5): 485–495, 1996.

54. Otoole P and Lombard M. Vitamin C and gastric cancer: supplements for some or fruit for all. *Gut* 39(3): 345–347, 1996.

55. Greenberg ER, Baron JA, Tosteson TD, et al. A clinical trial of antioxidant vitamins to prevent colorectal adenoma. *N Engl J Med* 331: 141–147, 1994.

56. Kushi L, Fee R, Sellers T, et al. Intake of vitamins A, C, and E and postmenopausal breast cancer: the Iowa Women's Health Study. *Am J Epidemiol* 144(2): 165–174, 1996.

57. Hunter DJ, Manson JE, Colditz GA, et al. A prospective study of the intake of vitamins C, E, and A and the risk of breast cancer. *N Engl J Med* 329(4): 234–240, 1993.

58. Eberlein-Konig B, et al. Protective effect against sunburn of combined systemic ascorbic acid (vitamin C) and d-alpha-tocopherol (vitamin E). *J Am Acad Dermatol* 38 (1): 45–48, 1998.

59. Covington R. (Ed.) 370–372, 1996.

60. Cooper KH, 150, 1994.

61. Covington R. (Ed.) 370–372, 1996.

62. Levine M, et al. Proceedings of the national academy of sciences 93 (8): 3704–3709, April 16, 1996.

63. Gerster H. No contribution of ascorbic acid to renal calcium oxalate stones. *Ann Nutr Metab* 41(5): 269–282, 1997.

64. Butterworth CE, Jr. Effect of folate on cervical cancer. Synergism among risk factors. *Ann N Y Acad Sci* 669: 293–299, 1992; Kim Y-I, et al. Folate, epithelial dysplasia, and colon cancer. *Proc Assoc Am Physicians* 107: 218–227, 1995; Tseng M, et al. Micronutrients and the risk of colorectal adenomas. *Am J Epidemiol* 144 (11): 1005–1014, 1996; Heimberger DC. Localized deficiencies of folic acid in aerodigestive tissues. *Ann N Y Acad Sci* 669: 87–96, 1992.

65. Hercberg S, et al. Background and rationale behind the SU.VI.MAX Study, a prevention trial using nutritional doses of a combination of antioxidant vitamins and minerals to reduce cardiovascular diseases and cancers. SUpplementation en VItamines et Mineraux AntioXydants Study. *Int J Vitam Nutr Res* 68 (1): 3–20, 1998.

66. Butterworth CE, Jr, et al. Oral folic acid supplementation for cervical dysplasia: a clinical intervention trial. *Am J Obstet Gynecol* 166(3): 803–809, 1992.

67. Butterworth CE, Jr., Hatch KD, Gore H, et al. Improvement in cervical dysplasia associated with folic acid therapy in users of oral contraceptives. *Am J Clin Nutr* 35(1): 73–82, 1982; Zarcone R, Bellini P, Carfora E, et al. Folic acid and cervix dysplasia. *Minerva Ginecol* 48: 397–400, 1996; Childers JM, Chu J, Voigt LF, et al. Chemoprevention of cervical cancer with folic acid: a phase III Southwest Oncology Group Intergroup study. *Cancer Epidemiol Biomarkers Prev* 4(2): 155–159, 1995; Butterworth CE, Jr, et al., 1992.

68. Orr J, et al. Nutritional status of patients with untreated cervical cancer I and II. *Am J Ob Gyn* 151: 625–635, 1985.

69. Giovannucci E, et al. Folate, methionine, and alcohol intake and risk of colorectal adenoma. *Journal National Cancer Institute* 85(11): 875–884, June 2, 1993; Folic acid may cut colon cancer by 33%. *Executive Health's Good Health Report* 30:1, 3, October 1993.

70. Covington R. (Ed.) 372–373, 1996.

71. Murray MT, 1996, 119.

72. Covington R. (Ed.) 372–373, 1996.

73. Covington R. (Ed.) 372–373, 1996.

74. Mawer EB, et al. Serum 1,25-dihydroxyvitamin D may be related inversely to disease activity in breast cancer patients with bone metastases. *J Clin Endocrinol Metab* 82 (1): 118–122, 1997.

75. Garland FC, et al. Geographic variation in breast cancer mortality in the United States: a hypothesis involving exposure to solar radiation. *Prev Med* 19(6): 614–622, Nov 1990; Key SW and Marble M. Studies link sun exposure to protection against cancer. *Cancer Weekly Plus* 5–6, November 17, 1997.

76. Martinez ME, et al. Calcium, vitamin D, and the occurrence of colorectal cancer among women. *J Natl Cancer Inst* 88(19): 1375–1382, 1996.

77. Kearney J, et al. Calcium, vitamin D, and dairy foods and the occurrence of colon cancer in men. *Am J Epidemiol* 143(9): 907–917, 1996.

78. James SY, et al. Effects of 1,25 dihydroxyvitamin D3 and its analogues on induction of apoptosis in breast cancer cells. *J Steroid Biochem Mol Biol* 58(4): 395–401, 1996.

79. Taylor JA, et al. Association of prostate cancer with vitamin D receptor gene polymorphism. *Cancer Res* 56 (18): 4108–4110, 1996; Douglas WC. Vitamin D scores again. Second Opinion 7: 7, 4–5 July 1997.

80. Covington R. (Ed.) 368–369, 1996.

81. Covington R. (Ed.) 368–369, 1996.

82. Covington R. (Ed.) 368–369, 1996.

83. Covington R. (Ed.) 386–387, 1996.

84. Leonard TK, et al. Nutrient intakes: cancer causation and prevention. *Prog Food Nutr Sci* 10(3–4): 237–277, 1986.

85. Yang CS, Research on esophageal cancer in China: a review. *Cancer Res* (8 Pt 1): 2633–2644, 1980.

86. Berg JW, et al. Proceedings: epidemiology of gastrointestinal cancer. *Proc Natl Cancer Conf* 7: 459–464, 1972.

87. Covington R. (Ed.) 386–387, 1996.

88. Murray MT, 1996, 218.

89. Covington R. (Ed.) 386–387, 1996.

90. Covington R. (Ed.) 379–380, 1996.

91. Martinez ME and Willett WC. Calcium, vitamin D, and colorectal cancer: a review of the epidemiologic evidence. *Cancer Epidemiol Biomarkers Prev* 7(2): 163–168, 1998; Kearney J, et al. Calcium, vitamin D, and dairy foods and the occurrence of colon cancer in men. *Am J Epidemiol* 143(9): 907–917, 1996.

92. Whiting SJ. Safety of some calcium supplements questioned. *Nutr Rev* 52(3): 95–97, 1994. Review.

93. Covington R. (Ed.) 379–380, 1996.

94. Alberts DS, et al. Randomized, double-blinded, placebo-controlled study of effect of wheat bran fiber and calcium on fecal bile acids in patients with resected adenomatous colon polyps. *J Natl Cancer Inst* 88(2): 81–92, 1996; Liebman B. *Nutrition Action Health Letter* 23(2): 2, 1996.

95. Covington R. (Ed.) 379–380, 1996.

96. Covington R. (Ed.) 379–380, 1996.

Chapter Six

1. Hall SS. *Health* 11: 3, 106–110, April, 1997.

2. Begley S, Springen K, et al. *Newsweek* 123: 17, 44–48, April 25, 1994.

3. Napier K. *Harvard Health Letter* 20: 6, 9–12, April 1995.

4. Di Mascio P, et al. Lycopene as the most efficient biological carotenoid singlet oxygen quencher. *Arch Biochem Biophysics* 274, 532–538, 1989.

5. Franceschi S, et al. Tomatoes and risk of digestive-tract cancers. *Int J Cancer* 59, 181–184, 1994.

6. Giovannucci E, et al. Intake of carotenoids and retinol in relation to risk of prostate cancer. *Journal National Cancer Institute* 87(23): 1767–1776, 1995; Marston W. Why pizza's better than ever. *Health* 12:1, 28–29, January/February 1998.

7. Zhang S, et al. Measurement of retinoids and carotenoids in breast adipose tissue and a comparison of concentrations in breast cancer cases and control subjects. *Am J Clin Nutr.* 66(3): 626–632, 1997.

8. Clinton SK, et al. Cis-trans lycopene isomers, carotenoids, and retinol in the human prostate. *Cancer Epidemiol Biomarkers Prev* 5(10): 823–833, 1996.

9. Kohlmeier L, et al. Lycopene and myocardial infarction risk in the EURAMIC Study. *Am J Epidemiol* 146(8): 618–626, 1997.

10. Day NE. Phyto-estrogens and hormonally dependent cancers. *Pathol Biol* 42(10): 1090, 1994.

11. Cline JM, et al. Phytochemicals for the prevention of breast and endometrial cancer. *Cancer Treat Res* 94: 107–134, 1998; Messina MJ, et al. Soy intake and cancer risk: a review of the in vitro and in vivo data. *Nutr Cancer* 21(2): 113–131, 1994.

12. Messina MJ, et al., 1994.

13. Barnes S, et al. Rationale for the use of genistein-containing soy matrices in chemoprevention trials for breast and prostate cancer. *J Cell Biochem Suppl* 22: 181–187, 1995; Magic beans. *Body Bulletin* 2, June 1995.

14. Messina MJ, et al., 1994.

15. Goodman MT, et al. Association of soy and fiber consumption with the risk of endometrial cancer. *Am J Epidemiol* 146(4): 294–306, 1997.

16. Ingram D, et al. Case-control study of phyto-oestrogens and breast cancer. *Lancet* 350 (9083): 990–994, 1997; Raloff J. Plant estrogens may ward off breast cancer. *Science News* 152: 15, 230, October 11, 1997.

17. Kaegi E. Unconventional therapies for cancer: 2. green tea. *CMAJ: Canadian Medical Association Journal* 158: 8, 1033–1035, 1998.

18. Katiyar SK and Mukhtar H. Tea antioxidants in cancer chemoprevention. *J Cell Biochem Suppl* 27: 59–67, 1997; Why green tea may help fight cancer. *Tufts University Health & Nutrition Letter* 15: 6, 2, August 1997.

19. Yang CS and Wang ZY. Tea and cancer. *Journal National Cancer Institute* 85(13): 1038–1049, 1993.

20. Khan SG, et al. Enhancement of antioxidant and phase II enzymes by oral feeding of green tea polyphenols in drinking water to SKH-1 hairless mice: Possible role in cancer chemoprevention. *Cancer Res* 52, 4050–4052, 1992.

21. Stich HF. Teas and tea components as inhibitors of carcinogen formation in model systems and man. *Prev Med* 21: 377–384, 1992.

22. Katiyar SK and Mukhtar H, 1997.

23. Wang ZY, et al. Inhibitory effects of black tea, green tea, decaffeinated black tea, and decaffeinated green tea on ultraviolet B light-induced skin carcinogenesis in 7,12-dimethylbenz[a]anthracene-initiated SKH-1 mice. *Cancer Res* 54(13): 3428–3435, 1994.

24. Imai K, et al. Cancer-preventive effects of drinking green tea among a Japanese population. *Prev Med* 26(6): 769–775, 1997.

25. Kohlmeier L, et al. Tea and cancer prevention: an evaluation of the epidemiologic literature. *Nutr Cancer* 27(1): 1–13,1997.

26. Ji BT, et al. Green tea consumption and the risk of pancreatic and colorectal cancers. *Int J Cancer* 70(3): 255–258, 1997.

27. Yu GP, et al. Green-tea consumption and risk of stomach cancer: a population-based case-control study in Shanghai, China. *Cancer Causes Control* 6 (6): 532–538, 1995.

28. Key SW and Marble M. Researchers to test green tea as cancer fighter. *Cancer Weekly Plus* 24–25, September 15, 1997.

29. Kaegi E, 1033–1035, 1998.

30. Kaegi E, 1033–1035, 1998.
31. Murray MT, 21–129, 261–263, 1995.
32. Pressing garlic for possible health benefits. *Tufts University Diet & Nutrition Letter* 12: 7, 3–6, September 1994.
33. Ip C, et al. Efficacy of cancer prevention by high-selenium garlic is primarily dependent on the action of selenium. *Carcinogenesis* 11, 2649–52, 1995.
34. Sumiyoshi H. New pharmacological activities of garlic and its constituents. *Nippon Yakurigaku Zasshi* 110 (Suppl 1): 93P–97P, Oct. 1997. Review; Agarwal KC. Therapeutic actions of garlic constituents. *Med Res Rev* 16(1): 111–124, 1996.
35. Steinmetz KA, et al. Vegetables, fruit and colon cancer in the Iowa Women's Health Study. *Am J Epidemiol* 139(1): 1–13, 1994.
36. Forkert PG, et al. Protection from 1,1-dichloroethylene-induced Clara cell injury by diallyl sulfone, a derivative of garlic. *J Pharmacol Exp Ther* 277(3): 1665–1671, 1996; Garlic: The aroma of wellness. *Maclean's* 110: 5, 62, February 3, 1997.
37. Fukushima S, et al. Cancer prevention by organosulfur compounds from garlic and onion. *J Cell Biochem Suppl* 27: 100–105, 1997.
38. Dorant E. Consumption of onions and a reduced risk of stomach carcinoma. *Gastroenterology* 110(1): 12–20, 1996.
39. Covington R. (Ed.) 702–703, 1996.
40. Murray MT, 261–263, 1995.
41. Covington R. (Ed.) 702–703, 1996.
42. Covington R. (Ed.) 702–703, 1996.
43. Murray MT, 1996.
44. Messina M and Barnes S. Phyto-oestrogens and breast cancer. *Lancet* 350: 9083, 971–972, 1997.
45. Serraino M, et al. The effect of flaxseed supplementation on the initiation and promotional stages of mammary tumorigenesis. *Nutr Cancer* 17(2): 153–159, 1992.
46. Ingram D, et al. Case-control study of phyto-oestrogens and breast cancer. *Lancet* 350 (9083): 990–994, 1997.
47. Bougnoux P, et al. Alpha-linolenic acid content of adipose breast tissue: a host determinant of the risk of early metastasis in breast cancer. *Br J Cancer* 70(2): 330–334, 1994.
48. Murray MT, 266–267, 1996.
49. Hunter BT. Could licorice prevent cancer? *Consumers' Research Magazine* 77:10, 8–9, October 1994; Murray MT, 228–238, 1995.
50. Arase Y. The long-term efficacy of glycyrrhizin in chronic hepatitis C patients. *Cancer* 79(8): 1494–1500, 1997.
51. Arase Y, 1997.
52. Murray MT, 228–238, 1995.
53. Arase Y, 1997.

54. Yun TK, et al. A case-control study of ginseng intake and cancer. *Int J Epidemiol* 19 (4): 871–876, 1990.

55. Covington R. (Ed.) 709, 1996; Tyler VE. What pharmacists should know about herbal remedies. *J APhA* NS36 (1): 29–37, 1996.

56. Ploss E and Meyer CA. Panax ginseng. scientific report. Cologne: Kooperation Phytopharmaka, 1988; Lawrence Review of Natural Products. Ginseng monograph, Facts and Comparisons Division, St. Louis, Missouri: JB Lipincott Company, March, 1990; Tyler V. Herbs of choice. New York: Haworth Press, 1994.

57. Tyler V. Herbs of choice. New York: Haworth Press, 1994; Schulz V, et al. Rational phytotherapy. New York: Springer-Verlag, 1998.

58. Covington R. (Ed.) 96, 1996.

59. Bogdanov IG, et al. Antitumor effect of glycopeptides from the cell wall of *Lactobacillus bulgaricus.* (Article in Russian). *Biull Eksp Biol Med* 84(12): 709–712, December 1977.

60. Aso Y, et al. Preventive effect of a *Lactobacillus casei* preparation on the recurrence of superficial bladder cancer in a double-blind trial. The BLP Study Group. *Eur Urol* 27(2): 104–109, 1995.

61. Dash SK. Acidophilus: The friendly bacteria. *Total Health* (April 4,) 17:2, 27–28, 1995.

62. Low dose medication will treat insomnia. *Psychopharmacology Update* 6:10, 3, October 1995.

63. Bartsch C and Bartsch H. Significance of melatonin in malignant diseases. *Wien Klin Wochenschr* (Article in German), 109(18): 722–729, October 3, 1997.

64. Molis TM, et al. Melatonin modulation of estrogen-regulated proteins, growth factors, and proto-oncogenes in human breast cancer. *J Pineal Res* 18(2): 93–103, 1995.

65. Panzer A. Melatonin in osteosarcoma: an effective drug? *Med Hypotheses* 48(6): 523–525, 1997.

66. Huang MT, et al. Inhibitory effects of curcumin on tumorigenesis in mice. *J Cell Biochem Suppl* 27: 26–34, 1997.

67. Huang MT, et al., 1997.

68. Murray MT, 162–171, 1995.

69. Kumazawa Y, et al. Activation of peritoneal macrophages by berberine-type alkaloids in terms of induction of cytostatic activity. *Int J Immunopharmacol* 6(6): 587–592, 1984.

70. Zhang RX, et al. Laboratory studies of berberine used alone and in combination with 1,3-bis(2-chloroethyl)-1-nitrosourea to treat malignant brain tumors. *Chin Med J* (Engl). 103(8): 658–665,1990.

71. Covington R. (Ed.) 708, 1996.

72. Covington R. (Ed.) 708, 1996.

73. Murray MT, 60–68, 1995.

74. Valstar E. Nutrition and cancer: A review of the preventive and therapeutic abilities of single nutrients. *Journal of Nutritional Medicine* 4:2, 179–198, 1994.

75. Murray MT, 60–68, 1995.

76. Murray MT, 60–68, 1995.

77. Fahey JW, et al. Broccoli sprouts: an exceptionally rich source of inducers of enzymes that protect against chemical carcinogens. *Proc Natl Acad Sci USA* 94(19): 10367–10372, 1997; Talalay P, et al. Chemoprotection against cancer by phase 2 enzyme induction. *Toxicol Lett* 82–83, 173–179, 1995.

78. Zhang Y, et al. A major inducer of anticarcinogenic protective enzymes from broccoli: isolation and elucidation of structure. *Proc Natl Acad Sci USA* 89(6): 2399–2403, 1992.

79. Jaret P. The newest cancer fighter. *Health* 12: 3, 26v27, April 1998.

80. Key SW and Marble M. Cancer protection compound abundant in broccoli sprouts. *Cancer Weekly Plus* 18–19, September 29, 1997.

81. Raloff J. Anticancer agent sprouts up unexpectedly. *Science News* 152: 12, 183, 1997.

82. Jang M, et al. Cancer chemopreventive activity of resveratrol, a natural product derived from grapes. *Science* 275 (5297): 218–220, Jan. 10, 1997; Key SW and Marble M. Grape compound may inhibit cancer. *Cancer Weekly Plus* 13–14, January 20, 1997.

83. Jang M, et al., 1997; Key SW and Marble M, 1997.

84. Key SW and Marble M. Compounds in milk may reduce early indicators of cancer. *Cancer Weekly Plus* 8, November 11, 1996.

85. Amagase H, et al. Dietary rosemary suppresses 7,12-dimethylbenz(a)anthracene binding to rat mammary cell DNA. *J Nutr* 126(5): 1475–1480, 1996; Key SW and Marble M. Rosemary may have anti-cancer properties. *Cancer Biotechnology Weekly* 9–10, June 3, 1996.

86. Key SW and Marble M. Researchers search for anti-cancer compounds in food. *Cancer Weekly Plus* 17, 1997.

87. Jaret P and Schrager V. Foods that fight cancer. *Health* 9: 2, 58–63, March/April 1995.

88. Knekt P, et al. Dietary flavonoids and the risk of lung cancer and other malignant neoplasms. *Am J Epidemiol* 146(3): 223–230, 1997; Babiarz L. An apple a day may keep lung cancer away. *Walking Magazine* 13: 2, 23, April 1998.

89. Breast cancer prevention. *Herizons* 11: 3, 10, Summer 1997.

90. Pisha E, et al. Discovery of betulinic acid as a selective inhibitor of human melanoma that functions by induction of apoptosis. *Nat Med* 1(10): 1046–1051, 1995; Centofanti M. Birch bark has an anticancer bite. *Science News* 148: 15, 231, October 7, 1995.

91. Zhao GX, et al. Asimin, asiminacin, and asiminecin: novel highly cytotoxic asimicin isomers from Asimina triloba. *J Med Chem* 37(13): 1971–1976, 1994; Grape and pawpaw may help fight cancer. *Futurist* 32: 3, 7, April 1998.

Chapter Seven

1. Shephard RJ. Exercise in the prevention and treatment of cancer. An update. *Sports Med* 15(4): 258–280, April 1993.
2. Martinez ME, et al. Leisure-time physical activity, body size, and colon cancer in women. Nurses' Health Study Research Group. *J Natl Cancer Inst* 89(13): 948–955, 1997; Franklin D and Henry S. Walk away from colon cancer. *Health* 11: 7, 16, October 1997.
3. Hills AP and Byrne NM. Exercise prescription for weight management. *Proc Nutr Soc* 57(1): 93–103, 1998; Pinto BM and Szymanski L. Exercise in weight management. *Med Health R I* 80(11): 361–363, November 1997.
4. Cooper KH, 47, 1994.
5. Lee IM, Paffenbarger RS, Jr. Physical activity and its relation to cancer risk: a prospective study of college alumni. *Med Sci Sports Exerc* 26(7): 831–837, July 1994.
6. Colditz GA, et al. Physical activity and reduced risk of colon cancer: implications for prevention. *Cancer Causes Control* 8(4): 649–667, 1997.
7. Osborne M, et al., 1997.
8. Thun MJ, et al. Alcohol consumption and mortality among middle-aged and elderly U.S. adults. *N Engl J Med* 11 337(24): 1705–1714, 1997.
9. Osborne M, et al., 1997.
10. Key SW and Marble M. More research suggests moderate tanning prevents cancer. *Cancer Weekly Plus* 18, Nov 25–Dec 2, 1996.
11. Tangley L and Gest T. Deadly rays may pierce the screen. *US News & World Report* 124: 8, 37, Mar. 2, 1998.
12. Osborne M, et al., 1997.
13. Winawer SJ and Shike M. *Cancer Free.* New York: Simon & Schuster, 158, 1995.
14. Campion EW. Power lines, cancer, and fear. *N Engl J Med* 337(1): 44–46, 1997; Electromagnetic fields from power lines don't cause cancer. *Consumers' Research Magazine* 80: 8, 7 August 1997.
15. Colditz GA. Hair dye and cancer: Reassuring evidence of no association. *Journal of the National Cancer Institute* 86: 3, 164–165, 1994.
16. Stress reduction may help our bodies defend against disease. *Women's Health Weekly* 9, January 12, 1998.

17. Longo D, 1998.
18. Andersen BL, et al. Stress and immune responses after surgical treatment for regional breast cancer. *Journal National Cancer Institute* 90(1): 30–36, 1998; Griffith K and Holmes B, et al. Can easing stress fight cancer? *Health* 12(3):15, April 1998.
19. Andersen BL, et al. Stress and immune responses after surgical treatment for regional breast cancer. *Journal National Cancer Institute* 90(1): 30–36, 1998.
20. Funk D. Military programs to tackle breast cancer head on. *Army Times* 58: 3, 18, August 18, 1997.

Index

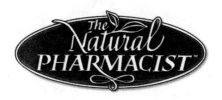

About the Author

Richard Harkness, Pharm., FASCP, an honors graduate of the Northeast Louisiana University School of Pharmacy, is a consultant pharmacist and a certified smoking cessation specialist. A nationally syndicated columnist, public speaker, and teacher, he is the author of *Drug Interactions Guide Book* (Prentice-Hall), *Drug Interactions Handbook* (Prentice-Hall), *OTC Handbook: What to Recommend & Why* (Medical Economics Co.), and *The Natural Pharmacist Guide to Heart Disease Prevention* (Prima).

About the Series Editors

Steven Bratman, M.D., medical director of Prima Health, has many years of experience in the alternative medicine field. A graduate of the University of California at Davis, Medical School, he has also trained in herbology, nutrition, Chinese medicine, and other alternative therapies, and has worked closely with a wide variety of alternative practitioners. He is the author of *The Natural Pharmacist: Your Complete Guide to Herbs* (Prima), *The Natural Pharmacist: Your Complete Guide to Illnesses and Their Natural Remedies* (Prima), *The Natural Pharmacist Guide to St. John's Wort and Depression* (Prima), *The Alternative Medicine Ratings Guide* (Prima), and *The Alternative Medicine Sourcebook* (Lowell House).

David J. Kroll, Ph.D., is a professor of pharmacology and toxicology at the University of Colorado School of Pharmacy and a consultant for pharmacists, physicians, and alternative practitioners on the indications and cautions for herbal medicine use. A graduate of both the University of Florida and the Philadelphia College of Pharmacy and Science, Dr. Kroll has lectured widely and has published articles in a number of medical journals, abstracts, and newsletters.